To Dr. Leonard I. Stein

my friend and teacher
for over twenty years.

Contents

Preface

This book started as a handout for a series of lectures on psychopharmacology I first gave in 1974 at the Santa Clara Valley Medical Center in California as a beginning psychiatry resident. At that time, non-physicians staff members, from nurses to social workers to psych techs, were not expected to be educated about medications.Though they spent considerable time sharing their experience and knowledge and had much more contact with the patients than did the physicians, they were discouraged from making suggestions about prescriptions and from monitoring the effects of medications. I began to realize that if these members of the treatment team knew what to look for, they could take on an important role in determining what medication might be useful, how well the medication was working, and what side effects were present. These lectures were my way of sharing information with people who had taught me and conveying my realization that medication decisions needed the input of the entire team of people working with the patient.

As patients have taken increasingly active roles in their own care, they have come to be recognized as clients or, more recently, consumers of mental health care. They, too, must be educated as much as possible. By 1987 I was regularly giving the psychopharmacology lectures for nonmedical staff. One of my own clients found the information extremely useful and asked why clients were not invited. My only response was that I had never thought about it. Since that time, I have invited clients to training sessions I give on psychopharmacology and other topics.

At times, this means that state hospital patients leave their inpatient units and go down to the lecture hall. The clients' questions and comments have added to the richness of the teaching, and so far no client has behaved inappropriately during a lecture.

Note that the best way to learn about psychopharmacology is to work with clients—information learned from a book or a lecture can be difficult to remember. The purpose of this book is to give you a sense of the different classes of medications, suggest some basic concepts about medications, and help you build your vocabulary. Your job is to get in the habit of learning about the medications your clients are taking. The way to remember the information in this book is to connect it to a real person. In this as in many other things, our clients are our best teachers.

Acknowledgments

Many people have helped with earlier drafts of this handout as it has been written, edited, and changed over the years. I would like to thank Marena Kehl for editing the first version of this more than 20 years ago, and Charlie Kargas and Nancy Salzwedel for their help reading through this year's update. I would particularly like to thank Peter Weiden for his many helpful comments on this draft.

Abbreviations

qd	once a day
bid	twice a day
tid	three times a day
qid	four times a day
hs	before bed
prn	as needed
po	by mouth
IM	intramuscular (injection)
IV	intravenous
STAT	right away
i	one unit or pill
ii	two units or pills
iii	three units or pills
c or q	with
s	without
CBC	complete blood count, including both red and white cell count

1

Psychopharmacology: The Rules of the Game

This book is a distilled and abridged version of my own views on the use of psychotropic medications. Medication is an increasingly important part of comprehensive mental health treatment. The nonmedical therapist often knows the client better than the physician does and therefore is often in the best position to help determine which medications may be helpful for a new client and to evaluate the effectiveness of medication a client is taking at the time.

Medication is often presented as an alternative to other forms of therapy, leading us to believe we must choose between competing options. The available research suggests just the opposite—that appropriately used medication can facilitate other therapy. Similarly, the appropriate use of psychosocial therapy can facilitate the effectiveness of medication, as well as increase the likelihood that the client will take the medication reliably. This is not to suggest that medications are effective for everyone or that they are not without risks and problems. It does suggest that all therapists, whether philosophically inclined toward biological treatment or not, need to be as knowledgeable as possible about the potential benefits and limitations of psychotropic medications.

This guide is not meant to be definitive in any sense. Only those classes of medications I believe are most important are covered, and theoretical issues are completely ignored. *It is important to keep in mind that the specific indications for use and the specific dosages given are only meant to be rough approx-*

imations that fit with my personal experience. If you are working with a client who is taking a medication with which you are unfamiliar, you can find information about the dosage, contraindications, and side effects in the *Physician's Desk Reference* (*PDR*) or some other recent medication reference.

While the information in this monograph comes primarily from the references cited at the end of this book, much of it also comes from other papers and books I have read over the years. It is not meant to be an academic treatise, and I have not documented the source for every idea presented.

Rules of the Game

1. *The five major classes of medications.* For most practical purposes, medications can be divided into five major classes. These include:

   - Antipsychotics
   - Side effect medications
   - Antidepressants
   - Mood stabilizers
   - Antianxiety medications

   These five categories include the vast majority of psychotropic prescriptions, which are enough to handle almost all common clinical problems.

   Within each class are a few different types of medications. For example, the antidepressants class includes SSRIs (selective serotonin reuptake inhibitors), tricyclics, and MAOIs (monoamine-oxidase inhibitors). Each type of medication is represented by many different specific medications, each with its own name. Medications of the same kind usually are much more similar than different. Therefore, learning about one or two medications in a class can help you understand the other medications in that class.

2. *Side effects/other actions.* All medications have at least some action in addition to the specific effect you want. For example,

in addition to having anti-pain properties, aspirin decreases the ability of the blood to form clots. Sometimes aspirin is used to decrease blood clotting; other times it is used as a pain reliever. Aspirin taken as a pain reliever has the potential to become life-threatening because of its anti-blood-clotting properties. Since medications have multiple effects, some of which are likely to be negative, you should not give a medication without a good reason.

3. *Drug-drug interactions.* Many medications that are very safe alone can be dangerous when taken in combination with other drugs. For example, many SSRI antidepressants can interfere with how tricyclic antidepressants are broken down and disposed of by the liver. Giving someone Prozac (an SSRI antidepressant) if he is on a stable dose of nortriptyline (a tricyclic antidepressant) can cause a dangerous buildup of the latter. Since Prozac stays in the body for a long time, rapidly switching someone from Prozac to nortriptyline can have the same effect if it is not done carefully. Furthermore, administering two different drugs that act on different parts of the serotonin system, such as the MAOI Parnate and the SSRI Zoloft, can cause an extremely dangerous serotonergic syndrome (fever, muscle jerking, confusion, rapid fluctuations of blood pressure and other autonomic systems).

4. *Other medications.* Always ask about *all* other medications the person is taking, both prescription and non-prescription. For example, many medications used to control high blood pressure can cause or exacerbate depression. Changing an offending medication may be much more effective than psychotherapy or adding another medication. Often people will not mention herbal remedies or birth control pills unless they are specifically asked.

5. *Other medical problems.* Ask about any medical problems the person has currently or has had in the past. We are in the business of treating the "whole person," and it is important to realize the extent to which medical illness and non-psychiatric

medications can influence mood and behavior.

6. *Allergic reactions.* Be aware that people can have an allergic reaction to any medication. Ask the client about medication allergies before any medication is prescribed.

7. *Names of medications.* Different medications often have very similar names. For example, Klonopin (clonazepam) is a benzodiazepine with anticonvulsant properties. Clonidine (Catapres) is an antihypertensive medication often used to help decrease the symptoms of narcotic and other drug withdrawal. Clozapine is a new antipsychotic medication, and clomipramine is an antidepressant medication that is effective in obsessive compulsive disorder. Every medication has a generic, or chemical, name as well as a brand name from each manufacturer. A particular medication will always have only one generic name, but if it is made by several pharmaceutical companies, each company will give the medication a different trade name. For example, desipramine is the generic name for a common antidepressant that is marketed by one company under the name Norpramin and by another company under the name Pertofrane. The *PDR* is a common reference that cross lists all of the generic and trade names for all prescription medications.

8. *No one knows everything.* The most important thing is to recognize what you do not know, and how to get help. At some point, everyone calls someone else for help. A nonmedical clinician may get help from a psychiatrist; a psychiatrist may refer to an expert psychopharmacologist. For more information about medication, refer to the resources listed in the bibliography.

Thoughts on the Client/Clinician/Psychiatrist Relationship

This is obviously a complicated topic that deserves an entire book in itself. The purpose of any medication should be to help the client taking the medication feel better, be more in control of his or her own life, and be more functional. This requires that the client be informed about medication issues and involved in medication decisions. Be he case manager or therapist, the nonmedical clinician typically spends much more time with the client, knows the client better, and knows more about how the client is functioning and feeling than the psychiatrist does. The more the clinician knows about what to expect from medications, how they might help, and what side effects to look for, the more he or she will be able to help educate and involve the client and make sure that the psychiatrist has the information needed to make an informed decision about medication. Specific target goals for what it is hoped a medication will accomplish cannot be developed in isolation.

The client, clinician, and psychiatrist must operate as a team, and to a large extent, medication decisions should be made jointly by that team. The psychiatrist has ultimate authority over what medication will be prescribed. In most cases, the client has ultimate authority over what medication he or she will decide to take. Next to the client him- or herself, the nonmedical clinician has the most information about how medication can be most useful and whether it has worked. Everyone on the team must be aware of the concerns and goals of the other team members. My strong preference is that medication assessments be made with both psychiatrist and nonmedical clinician participating in the assessment, sharing information with each other and with the client.

It is important to think about when and how much information should be shared. When working with a very anxious, frightened, or confused client who is not processing information well, focus on the information needed to make immediate decisions. Basic information about how the medication might help, ways for both clients and clinicians to determine if the medication is working, and common side effects of the medication should be discussed even with an acutely upset client. Giving too much information all at once to someone who is very upset can overload the person and actually get in the way of learning.

Over time, the clinician should initiate a more in-depth discussion of the risks and benefits, long-term side effects, and other issues about the medication so that the client can be an informed collaborator in his or her own treatment. Withholding information about side effects or alternative treatments is paternalistic and disrespectful; moreover, it interferes with the kind of long-term relationship-building that promotes effective treatment and helps the client make responsible decisions about his or her medication. Clinicians often fear that too much information about side effects may discourage a client from taking medication. My experience is that a frank, open, balanced discussion that includes clear explanation of both risks and benefits promotes long-term medication use. I use my own judgment to decide how quickly and how much information I should share, but my assumption is that over time I will provide as much information as possible. Some clinicians worry that clients will stop taking a medication if they are given too much information about side effects. If a client is determined to stop taking medication, information on side effects and benefits is unlikely to sway him one way or the other. In any case, sharing information in a straightforward way promotes a healthy relationship that is essential for regular medication use.

Communicating with Physicians

Nonmedical mental health professionals, such as social workers, have learned to communicate very differently than physicians have. Training for social work stresses knowing all aspects of the client's situation. When social workers talk with one another, they illustrate their competence by demonstrating that they know their clients very well. Their clinical descriptions tend to be rich in detail. Physicians, on the other hand, are trained to use data to make a decision quickly. When physicians talk with each other about a patient, they present a very tightly organized summary of the patient and the problem and leave out all information that is not directly relevant. This communication style is reinforced by the limited amount of time available for physicians to talk with each other.

Nonmedical staff often pass on information at treatment planning meetings or team meetings where there is at least some time set aside to talk about the client. Physicians, whether psychiatrists or other other physicians, often find themselves talking about a client in the brief gaps between patient visits, when there are only a few minutes to answer a couple phone calls or write a note. Time is precious, and the physician has learned to get to the point quickly.

Often, the physician sees the social worker's detailed descriptions as long, rambling, disorganized discussions that never really address what needs to be done immediately. The physician prefers one-line summaries of the most relevant information needed for an immediate decision. This can leave the social worker feeling like the physician is cold, disinterested, and does not really know the client very well.

Understanding these differences can help make communication easier. If a social worker wants to effectively communicate with a physician, he or she should try to organize the point being made, leave out extra detail, and be aware of any time limitations. If a physician wants to communicate with a social worker, he or she should use a less abbreviated style and value the richness of detail provided by the social worker.

Thoughts for the Client Who Is Taking Medication

Medication is a tool that may help you cope with mental illness. Modern medications are extremely effective in helping people live with many different kinds of mental illness, from anxiety disorders to depression to schizophrenia. Medications do not always work as well as we might hope, and they often have more side effects than we would like. Some people have a goal to take as little medication as possible or to get off medication as soon as possible. I personally feel that a better goal is to figure out how to use medication so that you can have a life as close to the one you would like as possible.

I think it is very important for anyone taking medications to get as much information about them as possible. Having some information can help you figure out what else you might want to ask your psychiatrist. It can help you to understand what kinds of side effects you might experience and to be realistic about how your medications can help. Finally, having more information can help you to make better decisions about whether you are willing to take the medications prescribed by your psychiatrist.

Clients often have many questions about their medication that they never ask. Sometimes they find it difficult to ask their psychiatrist questions, or there is not enough time to ask questions, or they feel intimidated, or they do not know how to put their questions into words. It is often helpful to write down questions so that you can remember them. Others find it helpful to practice with a friend or therapist what they want to say to the psychiatrist. Appointments with psychiatrists are often shorter than either you or the psychiatrist would like. It may not be possible to get all questions answered in one visit. Think about which questions are most important and which can be put off until your next visit.

The following ideas are important if you are going to be involved in decisions about your own medication.

1. *Make sure that you know what medication you are taking.* Ask the psychiatrist or nurse to write down the name of each medication, along with instructions about how you are supposed to take it.

2. *Make sure you know what each medication is supposed to do.* What symptoms is each supposed to help with? How long will it take to know the medication is helping?

3. *Think about how your symptoms are interfering with things*

you want to do. Are your symptoms interfering with having friends, getting a job, going shopping, enjoying things?

4. *Besides taking medication, what other things can you do to control your symptoms?* What have you tried? What has worked and what has not? Often there are lots of things that you can do to control symptoms and achieve your own goals. Medication may be an important part of this, but medication will work better if it is combined with other ways of controlling symptoms.
5. *Work with your psychiatrist and other clinicians to develop your own list of goals,* and then track whether the medication helps you achieve them. Are you better able to go shopping, or talk to people, or read a book since you began taking the medication? Involve your psychiatrist in your goals. What do you want from your medication?
6. Make sure that your psychiatrist is aware of any medication side effects. Some side effects, like the restlessness that some people get with antipsychotic medication, are extremely difficult to live with. Other side effects, like the sexual problems caused by a number of antipsychotic and antidepressant medications, may be embarrassing to talk about. Your psychiatrist cannot help with these side effects if he or she is not aware of them.

Taking Medication Regularly

Most people with chronic illness do not take their medication as prescribed by their doctor. This is just as true for people with chronic medical illness as it is for people with chronic mental illness. This is sometimes addressed as a problem with medication "compliance," but the word "compliance" assumes that the client should comply or blindly follow the prescription of the physician. Ideally, the client-doctor relationship is collaborative, and the goal is to work with the client so that he or she takes the medication in a way that maximizes its effectiveness and minimizes its side effects. This typically means taking medication regularly.

This again deserves an entire book, but there are a few short hints that can be used.

1. *Simplify the medication-taking routine.* The more different bottles that must be opened and the more different times of day that medication must be taken, the less likely the medication will be taken reliably. People are fairly reliable about taking a medication once a day. It is harder for most people to take medication twice a day, and almost impossible for most people to take medication reliably three or four times a day. Most medications used in psychiatry can be taken once a day, including lithium and antipsychotics. Work with the physician to simplify the medication regiment whenever possible.
2. *Arrange for medication to be taken along with some other regular activity.* Taking medication with breakfast or when brushing one's teeth makes it easier to remember.
3. *Arrange packaging* that helps remind the person to take his or her medication. Plastic containers that allow the person to load a week's worth of medication into compartments labeled by the day of the week can help. At times we have made arrangements with our local pharmacy to package medication in individual plastic envelopes, one for each time a medication should be taken. For example, a person taking four different medications simply takes the medication in the "Monday morning" envelope. This eliminates the need to keep track of different numbers of pills from several pill bottles.
4. *Pay attention to side effects.* Even subtle side effects that are unrecognized and untreated can lead a client to decide to discontinue medication. Akasthisia, the motor restlessness that comes from some antipsychotic medications, is extremely uncomfortable, and clients often stop taking medication because of it.

5. *Be interested in the person's medication use.* Ask what medications the person is taking. View changes the person has made in medication use as the beginning of a conversation, rather than as an indication the person has done something wrong. If someone decides to take more or less medication, ask how he or she made that decision. Most client-initiated medication changes are not just accidents or figments of some psychotic process. To be useful, we must understand the client's decision-making process.
6. *Connect the medication in concrete ways to the person's own life goals.* If getting a job is what the person wants most, he is going to be more willing to take medication if he believes that taking the medication really will help him get a job.
7. *Arrange for medication to be supervised* when necessary. A person who is willing but regularly forgets to take medication can be helped by regular phone calls, or by visits from a clinician if mobile outreach services are available.

Before Starting Any Medication

1. *A diagnosis needs to be made first.* Medications should not be given just because a client is upset or even because he or she is psychotic. It is necessary first to become clear about the entire situation.

   Corollary A: Delirium needs to be ruled out first. Delirium is easily confused with psychosis but can be distinguished by a careful mental status exam. Clients with delirium are often disoriented and almost always have memory impairment.

   Corollary B: Medical illness or drug intoxication needs to be considered, as these may present as psychosis.
2. *A medication history needs to be obtained* (what medications the client has taken in the past, in what doses, with what effects). If a client previously has had a good response to a particular medication, it makes sense to restart that same drug.

3. *Follow treatment by picking out specific target symptoms and target goals.* Auditory hallucinations might be a target symptom for one client, disorganized thinking for another client, and social withdrawal for yet another. Functional goals are also extremely useful in helping connect medication to real life changes. Monitoring a client's ability to get out of his or her apartment more often, or to read, or to go grocery shopping may be a very useful way of understanding what kind of impact the medication is having on the person's life.
4. *Medications should be adjusted according to target symptoms and side effects.*
5. *More is not necessarily better.* Too much of most medications can cause an increase in side effects without necessarily being any more effective. Side effects can make the client's clinical symptoms worse, and at times drug side effects are difficult to distinguish from the illness being treated. Most medications take days or weeks to work. Increasing the dose because the client has not responded in the first 24 hours can lead to inappropriately high doses. At the same time, too low a dose of medication can prolong the discomfort and disability.
6. *Actively look for side effects.* Most medications make the person taking them uncomfortable, and all have side effects. Make sure the client knows about possible side effects before starting a new medication. Actively monitoring and treating side effects will help clients feel more comfortable and will also increase the client's willingness to continue taking the medications.

Laboratory Monitoring for People Taking Psychotropic Medications

The laboratory monitoring sections in this book all indicate what I believe to be the *minimal* requirement for monitoring a relatively young, healthy person with no complications who is in the community rather than a hospital. It takes into account the reality that most people dislike blood tests and that requiring too many will markedly decrease compliance. It also takes into account that we are often working with people with no insurance and little money.

If Medication Does Not Work

The medications used in psychiatry are generally as effective as any of the medications used in the rest of medicine. An antidepressant is as likely to help someone who is suffering from major depression as an antibiotic is to help someone with pneumonia. No medication in any field of medicine works 100% of the time.

As with many of the medications used in physical illness, psychiatric medications control symptoms, relieve pain, and preserve function, but do not cure the underlying condition. This can be frustrating, but it is common with most psychiatric and nonpsychiatric medications.

If medication does not work:

1. *Is the diagnosis correct?* Treatment is unlikely to work if the wrong thing is being treated. Correcting someone's biological predisposition to depression is less likely to be effective if the person is being overwhelmed by social stresses.
2. *Has a medical illness gone unrecognized?* The most conservative estimate is that 10% of psychiatric patients have unrecognized medical illnesses that are causing or contributing to their mental disorder.
3. *Is substance abuse interfering?* All of the common psychiatric symptoms can be caused or made worse by alcohol, stimulants, or other drugs.
4. *Is the person taking the medication?* Estimates are that half of all patients do not take medications as prescribed. A medication is unlikely to work if it is not being taken.
5. *Has the dose been high enough for a long enough period of time?* Almost all of the medications used in psychiatry take

days to weeks to be effective. Some medications such as clozapine can take months. Too often clients quit taking the medication before it has had a chance to work. Many clients who are "non-responders" go from one medication to another without giving any of them enough time to see if they would be effective. In other cases, a person will have stayed on a medication long enough but is taking such a low dose that it is unlikely to help.

The Basics of Psychopharmacology

Basic Classification of Psychotropic Medications

I. *Antipsychotic Agents* (these are sometimes referred to as neuroleptics or major tranquilizers, but they usually are not the best choice if the goal is tranquilization).

   A. traditional neuroleptics
      1. phenothiazines
         a. most sedating; e.g., chlorpromazine (Thorazine), thioridazine (Mellaril)
         b. least sedating; e.g., fluphenazine (Prolixin), trifluoperazine (Stelazine)
      2. butyrophenones; e.g., haloperidol (Haldol)
      3. thioxanthenes; e.g., thiothixene (Navane)
      4. miscellaneous traditional neuroleptics
         a. molindone (Moban)
         b. loxapine (Loxitane)
      5. long-acting injections; e.g., fluphenazine decanoate (Prolixin Decanoate) and haloperidol decanoate (Haldol Decanoate)

   B. atypical antipsychotics
      1. clozapine (Clozaril)
      2. risperidone (Risperdal)
      3. olanzapine (Zyprexa)
      4. quetiapine (Seroquel)

5. ziprasidone (Zeldox) (scheduled for release in summer 1998)

II. *Side Effect Medications—Antiparkinsonian Medications* (these are used to counteract the extrapyramidal, or muscle-related, side effects of traditional antipsychotic medications).

A. anticholinergic; e.g., benztropine (Cogentin)

B. diphenhydramine (Benadryl)

C. amantadine (Symmetrel)

III. *Antidepressants*

A. selective serotonin reuptake inhibitors (SSRIs); e.g., fluoxetine (Prozac) and sertraline (Zoloft)

B. miscellaneous "new-generation" antidepressants; e.g., trazodone (Desyrel), nefazodone (Serzone), and bupropion (Wellbutrin)

C. tricyclic antidepressants; e.g., desipramine (Norpramin) and nortriptyline (Pamelor)

D. monoamine oxidase inhibitors (MAOIs); e.g., phenelzine (Nardil) and tranylcypromine (Parnate)

IV. *Mood Stabilizers*

A. lithium (Eskalith, Lithane)

B. carbamazepine (Tegretol)

C. valproic acid (Depakote)

D. miscellaneous "new-generation" anticonvulsants; e.g., lamotrigine (Lamactil) and gabapentin (Neurontin)

V. *Antianxiety Medications and Sleeping Pills*

A. Antianxiety

1. benzodiazepines; e.g., diazepam (Valium) and alprazolam (Xanax)
2. buspirone (Buspar), a new anxiolytic that is unique in that it is supposed to be non-sedating and non-addicting.

3. meprobamate (Equanil, Miltown), barbiturates, and other older medications

B. Sleeping pills

1. zolpidem (Ambien) is a new non-benzodiazepine sleeping pill
2. benzodiazepines; e.g., temazepam (Restoril)
3. sedative antihistamines; e.g., diphenhydramine (Benadryl)
4. chloral hydrate

VI. *Miscellaneous*

A. beta-blockers; e.g., propranolol (Inderal)

B. stimulants; e.g., methylphenidate (Ritalin) and amphetamines (Dexadrine)

C. medications to decrease alcohol abuse

1. disulfiram (Antabuse)
2. naltrexone (ReVia)

How Do Drugs Work?

Most psychotropic drugs affect the activity of the brain by increasing or decreasing the activity of various *neurotransmitters*, chemical messengers that operate between adjacent nerve cells. A neurotransmitter is released when the axon terminal of a presynaptic neuron is excited. The substance then travels across the synapse to act on the target cell to either excite or inhibit it. Each neurotransmitter operates in multiple places in the brain, causing many different effects. More than 20 neurotransmitters have been identified. The important ones in psychopharmacology are *acetylcholine, dopamine, epinephrine, norephinephrine,* and *serotonin.*

Acetylcholine. This is a neurotransmitter widely present throughout the body. Acetylcholine receptors are called cholinergic receptors, and medications that block the action of acetylcholine by blocking receptors are called anticholinergic. The cholinergic system controls such things as salivation, gut motility, and the lens in the eye. Therefore, medications that block the cholinergic system typically cause dry mouth, blurred vision, and constipation. Anticholinergic medications can also cause memory problems, confusion, and delirium.

Dopamine/dopaminergic. This is a neurotransmitter found in the brain. A number of different dopamine receptors now have been identified. Traditional antipsychotic medications block the action of dopamine at the receptor sites in the receiving cells. Specifically, they block the D2 receptors in the mesolimbic part of the brain. Dopamine blockage seems to cause both the clinical effectiveness and the motor side effects of these medications. The "atypical" antipsychotic medications selectively block other dopamine receptors and non-dopamine receptors.

Epinephrine. This is the same as adrenaline. There are two kinds of adrenergic receptors: alpha and beta. Beta-blockers (propranolol) block the beta set of these receptors, leaving the alpha set intact.

Norepinephrine. Sometimes called noradrenalin, this neurotransmitter seems involved in depression and the ability to have positive feelings. Most antidepressants affect either norepinephrine or serotonin in complicated ways. The old, simplistic belief was that antidepressants blocked the deactivation of these neurotransmitters, effectively increasing the amount available. This view is too simple and probably inaccurate.

Serotonin. Abbreviated 5-HT for 5-hydroxytryptamine, this neurotransmitter is involved in depression, psychosis, and obsessive compulsive disorder. An increasing number of newer medications target different parts of this very complicated neurotransmitter system. There are now some 15 known kinds of serotonin receptors.

A Discussion About Time

Everything, including modern medicine, takes time, and clients often give up on medications or physicians change doses before the medication has had time to stabilize. Understanding the time a medication needs to take effect is an important part of developing a successful treatment plan. Often, the decision to use one medication rather than another is influenced by how quickly the medication works, or how long or short a period of time it stays in the person's body.

Absorption

A medication takes time to enter the bloodstream. An intravenous injection shows up in the blood immediately, while a pill taken on a full stomach may take an hour or more. Even after a medication is in the blood, it may take some time to cross the "blood-brain barrier" and enter the brain where it can take effect. Some medications are absorbed much more rapidly than others. Once absorbed, some medications cross into the brain more rapidly than others. Valium, for example, enters the brain very rapidly, while a similar medication like Serax may take somewhat longer. Benzodiazepines like Valium work almost immediately once they are in the brain. Most other psychotropic medications, including all antipsychotic and antidepressant medications, may take weeks to work even after a therapeutic level has been achieved. While the absorption time may influence how long it takes for a medication to work, more often other variables have much more impact.

Half-life

When a person takes the first dose of a new medication, the serum level goes up as the medication is absorbed and then falls as the medication is broken apart (metabolized) or gotten rid of (excreted). If a person takes a second dose of the medication before all of the previous dose has left the body, the second dose will add to the remaining part of the first dose. Most medications are eliminated slowly enough that the serum level continues to increase over time, even if the client takes the same dose of medication every day. The ups and downs eventually level off at what is called a "steady state serum level." If the person then stops taking the medication, the serum level of the medication will fall over time.

Half-life refers to how long it will take for half of the medication to leave the person's body. If a medication's half-life is 12 hours, half of the amount taken will be out of the body at the end of 12 hours; half of that amount (75% of the original dose) will be out after 24 hours; and half of that (87.5% of the original dose) will be out after 36 hours. It takes approximately five half-lives for a medication that is taken regularly to reach steady state. If a medication has a half-life of 24 to 100 hours (such as Dalmane), and is taken every night as a sleeping pill, the serum level of the medication will continue to increase every day for 5 to 20 days before steady state is reached. If a medication has a 10- to 20-day half-life (such as fluphenazine decanoate), and is given on a regular basis, the serum level of that medication will continue to increase over 50 to 100 days.

FIGURE 1.
Example of a 12-hour half-life

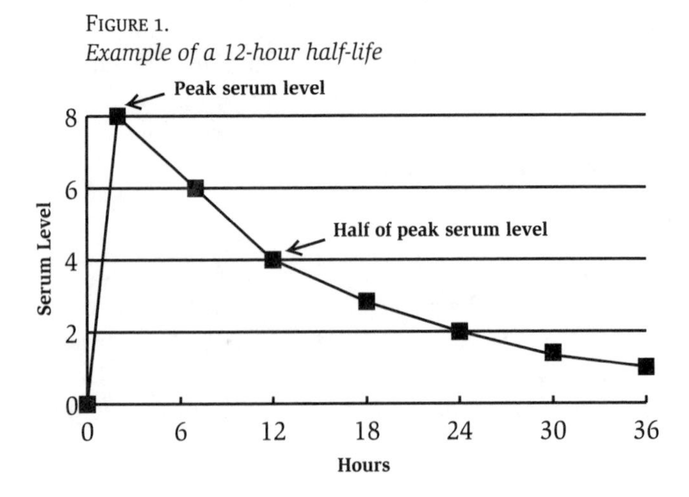

Time to Take Effect

Even after there is an effective serum level, it takes time for most psychotropic medications to work. It takes up to several weeks for most antidepressants to take effect, and if a client does not understand this, he or she may become frustrated by the lack of improvement and discontinue the medication shortly after it is started. Similarly, a client who is psychotic is often started on a moderate dose of an antipsychotic medication, but if the client does not improve within a few days, the dose is often increased. The dose of antipsychotic medication may be increased several times during the first week. Often, when the client then begins to respond to this higher dose, it is often mistakenly assumed that the client needs the higher dose. While that may be true, it is just as likely that the client simply needed time to respond and would have responded whether or not the dose was raised.

The opposite occurs when someone stops or decreases the dose of a medication. The serum level may drop in hours or days, but it may take weeks or even months for the person to get the full impact of the change. For example, many people with schizophrenia will not immediately become more symptomatic if they stop taking their antipsychotic medication, but they will be at a much higher risk for relapse over the next few weeks or months. In most cases, especially when a medication has been taken for a long time, one should wait weeks to months after decreasing the dose before making the next decrease.

Drug-Drug Interactions

There is increasing understanding of how one medication can affect other medications. In some cases, one medication can increase the effectiveness of another. For example, lithium sometimes is used to increase the effectiveness of an antidepressant. Similarly, one medication can increase the side effects of another. For example, antihistamines like diphenhydramine (Benadryl) can increase the tiredness, dry mouth, and constipation caused by tricyclic antidepressants like amitriptyline (Elavil).

Much recent interest has focused on how one drug can either increase or decrease how rapidly another medication is broken apart and deactivated by the body. For example, carbamazepine (Tegretol) *induces* (increases the activity of) the liver enzyme that metabolizes many other medications, including antipsychotic medications. As a result, if a person already taking an antipsychotic medication starts taking carbamazepine, his or her antipsychotic serum level will go down. Women taking oral contraceptives and carbamazepine are at greater risk for an unexpected pregnancy, because carbamazepine lowers the hormone level established by the oral contraceptives. Cigarette smoking induces the enzymes responsible for the metabolism of many antipsychotic medications, including clozapine and olanzapine, which in turn decreases the serum level of these medications.

On the other hand, fluoxetine (Prozac) interferes with the metabolism (and therefore raises serum levels) of many medications, including desipramine and diazepam (Valium). If not carefully monitored, a person taking fluoxetine along with a traditional antidepressant like desipramine (Pertofrane) can rapidly develop a dangerously high serum level of the traditional antidepressant. Fluoxetine has a very long half-life (7-9 days, including its active metabolite) so a significant amount of the medication can stay in a person's body for several weeks. When someone switches from fluoxetine to another antidepressant, the fluoxetine remaining after the switch can cause a rapid, potentially dangerous buildup of the new medication, unless there is a medication-free period of several weeks or the new medication is started at an extremely low dose.

While some of these interactions are relatively inconsequential, some may be life-threatening. For example, several antidepressants, including fluoxetine, can interfere with the metabolism of the non-sedating antihistamine terfenadine (Seldane), causing a life-threatening arrhythmia (irregular heart beat). Many of the most important drug-drug interactions center around the newer antidepressants and they will be discussed in more detail in that section. Drug-drug interactions affect many different medications, however, and it is one of the areas of psychopharmacology that is most complicated and is changing most rapidly.

Call a pharmacy if you have a question about possible drug-drug interactions. Most pharmacies have constantly updated references and computer programs that can be used to check the interactions between the various medications a person may be taking. Most pharmacies are glad to look up drug interactions even if the person is not receiving all of his or her medication from that pharmacy.

Drug-Drug Interactions and the P450 Enzyme System

The CYP450 enzymes are a collection of enzymes found in the liver that break down and deactivate a large number of substances, including medications and some foods. They are described by a number followed by a letter followed by another letter, for example, 1A2 and 2D6. The first number refers to the gene family, the letter refers to the gene subfamily, and the last letter refers to the specific gene number. The mechanisms of these enzymes are still being worked out, and only a few seem relevant to psychopharmacology.

A particular medication can induce (increase the activity) of an enzyme, or inhibit (decrease the activity) of an enzyme. A substrate is any medication or any other substance broken apart by a particular enzyme. (Note that Tables 1 and 2 do not cover all possible interactions.)

A Brief Discussion about Money

Those of us who prescribe, administer, and monitor psychotropic medications rarely consider how much they cost. Our clients, especially those who pay for their own medications, are painfully aware of the costs. The money spent on the medication is well worth it when measured against the increased suf-

Table 1. *Examples of Medications that Inhibit Specific P450 Enzymes Required for the Metabolism of Other Medications*

Relative Ranking	CYP 1A2	CYP 2C	CYP 2D6	CYP 3A3/4
Causes significant inhibition	fluvoxamine grapefruit juice	fluvoxamine fluoxetine	paroxetine fluoxetine sertraline	fluoxetine nefazodone
Relative Ranking	**CYP 1A2**	**CYP 2C**	**CYP 2D6**	**CYP 3A3/4**
Causes moderate to low inhibition	amitriptyline fluoxetine (high dose) imipramine paroxetine (high dose)	sertraline	secondary TCAs	sertraline tricyclic antidepressants
Causes minimal inhibition	bupropion mirtazapine nefazodone sertraline venlafaxine	venlafaxine	bupropion fluvoxamine mirtazapine nefazodone sertraline venlafaxine	mirtazapine paroxetine venlafaxine

Adapted from "Current Psychotropic Dosing and Monitoring Guidelines," by L. Ereshefsky, G. P. Overman, and J. K. Karp, July 1996, *Primary Psychiatry* 3(7), p. 26, by permission of *Primary Psychiatry*; and from "Practical Tips in Combining Antidepressants with Other Medications," by S. M. Stahl, 1996, American Psychiatric Association Symposium.

fering and dysfunction that would result if the medication were not available. Still, I think that we need to become more aware of the financial burden a prescription can impose. Often, less expensive alternatives are just as effective as newer, brand name medications. There is an unresolved debate about whether generic medications are as good as brand name medications. When I am prescribed medication by my physician, I generally use generic medications when they are available. However, some people report problems when switched from the brand name to the generic version of the same medication. Table 3 gives prices of common psychotropic medications in brand and generic froms. As you can see, it is very common for clients to be prescribed medication that costs more than $100 per month.

TABLE 2. *Examples of Medications Metabolized by Specific Enzymes (and that would have a rise in blood level if the enzyme were specifically inhibited)*

CYP 1A2	CYP 2C	CYP 2D6	CYP 3A3/4
acetaminophen	ibuprofen	chlorpheniramine	alprazolam
amitriptyline	diazepam	codeine (becomes ineffective)	clonazepam
caffeine	naproxen	desipramine	diazepam
clozapine	phenytoin	dextromethorphan	estrogen
haloperidol	propranolol	fluoxetine	steroids
imipramine	warfarin	haloperidol	carbamazepine
phenacetin	tolbutamide	hydrocodone	zolpidem
phenothiazines		nortriptyline	terfenadine (Serzone) can increase to lethal levels
theophylline		paroxetine	
		phenothiazines	
		propranolol	
		risperidone	
		venlafaxine	

Adapted from "Current Psychotropic Dosing and Monitoring Guidelines," by L. Ereshefsky, G. P. Overman, and J. K. Karp, July 1996, *Primary Psychiatry* 3(7), p. 26, by permission of *Primary Psychiatry*; and from "Practical Tips in Combining Antidepressants with Other Medications," by S. M. Stahl, 1996, American Psychiatric Association Symposium.

TABLE 3. *Prices of Common Psychotropic Medications*

Prices shown are based on average wholesale + $5.00 for brand name medications, and the maximum allowable price paid by Medicaid for generic medications. Prices may vary from one pharmacy to another.

	Quantity (Tablet Size x Average Number/day x 30 days)	Brand Name Typical dose for one month	Generic Typical dose for one month
ANTIPSYCHOTIC MEDICATIONS			
clozapine (Clozaril)*	100 mg x 4/day	$ 415.40	—
chlorpromazine (Thorazine)	100 mg x 4/day	$ 111.32	$ 26.36
fluphenazine (Prolixin)	10 mg/day	$ 63.07	$ 20.08
haloperidol (Haldol)	10 mg/day	$ 62.17	$ 6.22
loxapine (Loxitane)	25 mg x 4/day	$ 195.99	$ 112.92
molindone (Moban)	25 mg x 4/day	$ 163.64	$ 112.92
olanzapine (Zyprexa)	15 mg/day	$ 389.52	—
risperidone	2 mg x 2/day	$ 209.60	—
thioridazine (Mellaril)	100 mg x 4/day	$ 80.67	$ 28.40

	Quantity (Tablet Size x Average Number/day x 30 days)	Brand Name Typical dose for one month	Generic Typical dose for one month
ANTIPSYCHOTIC MEDICATIONS *continued*			
thiothixene (Navane)	20 mg/day	$ 50.90	$ 26.16
trifluoperazine (Stelazine)	20 mg/day	$ 122.29	$ 97.69
*plus week prescribing fee & weekly WBC			
(Long-acting injections)			
fluphenazine decanoate	12.5 mg x 2/month	$ 25.72	$ 16.64
haloperidol decanoate	100 mg/month	$ 55.90	—
ANTIDEPRESSANT MEDICATIONS			
amitriptyline (Elavil, Endep)	150 mg /day	$ 21.19	$ 7.09
bupropion (Wellbutrin)	100 mg x 3/day	$ 79.66	—
clomipramine (Anafranil)	75 mg x 2/day	$ 98.84	$ 78.36
desipramine (Norpramin, Pertofrane)	75 mg x 2/day	$ 98.20	$ 12.45
doxepin (Adapin, Sinequan)	100 mg x 2/day	$ 76.12	$ 11.75
fluoxetine (Prozac)	20 mg/day	$ 72.51	—
imipramine (Tofranil)	150 mg/day	$ 76.80	$ 7.77
mirtazapine (Remeron)	15 mg x 2/day	$ 123.80	—
nefazodone (Serzone)	200 mg x 2/day	$ 63.14	—
nortriptyline (Aventyl, Pamelor)	75 mg/day	$ 91.47	$ 12.45
paroxetine (Paxil)	20 mg/day	$ 66.92	—
sertraline (Zoloft)	100 mg/day	$ 69.67	—
trazodone (Desyrel)	100 mg x 3/day	$ 235.47	$ 47.80
venlafaxine (Effexor)	75 mg x 2/day	$ 77.98	—

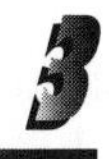

Antipsychotic Medications

These medications are sometimes referred to a "major tranquilizers." This is a misleading term. While these medications all have sedating and calming effects, their major effect is to reduce psychotic thinking and behavior. In general, other medications are safer and more effective if sedation is the sole aim. The term "neuroleptic" is also used for this class of medication, but this actually refers to a decrease in spontaneous and complex behaviors, which is a side effect rather than a positive effect of these medications.

Traditional Antipsychotic Medications

All of the older or traditional antipsychotic medications work by blocking receptor sites in the brain that are usually stimulated by a neurotransmitter called dopamine. Nerve cells communicate with each other by releasing chemicals called neurotransmitters, which are then picked up by receptors in the receiving nerve cell. Many neurotransmitters have now been discovered, including dopamine. Dopamine occurs in several different parts of the brain, and this dopamine receptor blockade accounts for many of the side effects of the medications as well as for their therapeutic actions.

All of the traditional antipsychotic medications are equally effective, but they vary in potency. That is, they all do an equally good job, but it takes different amounts of each medication for them to be equally effective. A 100 mg dose of Thorazine is equal in effectiveness to approximately 2 mg of Prolixin.

The different antipsychotic medications do have somewhat different side effects, although this is a matter of degree rather than kind. The high-potency medications are relatively less sedating, cause fewer anticholinergic side effects (anticholinergic refers to a medication that blocks the cholinergic part of the nervous system) such as dry mouth, constipation, and blurred vision, and cause less postural hypotension (drop in blood pressure from sitting down or standing up suddenly). They are also somewhat safer than low-potency medications. However, they more commonly cause extrapyramidal, or motor, side effects (EPSE), such as tremor and motor restlessness. Frequently, another medication (e.g., Cogentin), which may have its own side effects, is required to treat the extrapyramidal side effects.

In general, the high-potency antipsychotic medications (such as Prolixin, Haldol, and Navane) are both safer and better tolerated by most clients than low-potency medications such as Thorazine. This is especially true for paranoid clients, who may respond to the more sedating medications by feeling that they are losing control, which further frightens them.

Finally, when a medication is needed in an emergency, 5-10 mg IM (intramuscular) of Haldol or Prolixin hydrochloride is safe and has much more antipsychotic effect than 50-75 mg of IM chlorpromazine, which is the largest safe IM dose of that medication (note that both Haldol and Prolixin are available in a slow-onset, long-lasting decanoate injection that takes effect over days and lasts for weeks, and in a fast-onset, short-acting HCL or hydrochloride injection). Liquid medication works much faster than pills, almost as fast as injectable medication, and is generally preferred by the client. If additional sedation is needed, a benzodiazepine such as lorazepam can be given along with an antipsychotic medication.

Atypical Antipsychotic Medications

There are now several newer or "atypical" antipsychotic medications. I usually recommend one of these newer antipsychotic medications over the older, traditional medications for most people who need to start an antipsychotic or switch medications. I am cautious about switching medications for someone doing well on a traditional antipsychotic, but this can make sense for some people.

Clozapine was the first of these new-generation antipsychotic medications to be marketed. Risperidone (Risperdal) was released in February 1994, olanzapine (Zyprexa) in 1996, and quetiapine (Seroquel) in 1997. Several others are expected to be released in 1998. We now know there are at least five different dopamine receptors in the brain. All of the traditional antipsychotic medications (like haloperidol) work by blocking one kind of dopamine receptor called the D2 receptor. The atypical antipsychotic medications block a range of different dopamine receptors in addition to D2, the most important of which are the serotonin receptors. At this time, it is unclear which of the other dopamine receptors and which of the serotonin receptors are most important. Each of the new atypical antipsychotic medications has its own patterns of dopamine and serotonin blockade, and it may turn out that different patients will respond to different medications. Currently, data on this are very scarce.

All of these atypical antipsychotic medications have fewer extrapyramidal side effects than traditional medications. These medications also seem less likely to cause tardive dyskinesia. Furthermore, they appear to be more effective than the older medications. For example, clozapine is effective in many clients who have not responded to other antipsychotic medications. In addition, clozapine seems much more effective in treating "negative symptoms" (lack of motivation, flat affect) than traditional medications. The research is less complete on the other atypical medications, but it seems that these newer medications share clozapine's increased effectiveness on negative symptoms and ability to be effective with some people who have not responded to traditional antipsychotic medications. Finally, many people develop what is called a "dysphoric response," or feeling "zombie like," a few days after starting a traditional antipsychotic medication. They feel terrible but may not be able to describe it specifically. This response seems much less common with the new atypical medications.

Indications for Use

As noted before, a diagnosis should be made before starting any medication. Medications should not be given just because a client is upset or even because he or she is psychotic. Delirium needs to be ruled out first. In addition, medical illness or drug intoxication need to be considered, as these may present as psychosis.

1. *Psychosis.* When a psychotic client first takes an antipsychotic medication, there is an immediate calming effect that makes many clients more comfortable and decreases management problems. There is also a direct antipsychotic effect that takes several days or weeks to become evident; it can take weeks or months to see the full effect of an antipsychotic medication. In the past, clients with a diagnosis of schizophrenia who became psychotic and agitated were sometimes given Prolixin or Haldol in doses of 5-10 mg of liquid concentrate, pills, or by hourly injections until they calmed down. Recent research suggests that lower doses of these medications are usually as effective in decreasing psychotic symptoms as this "rapid neuroleptization" with administration of high-dose medication, while causing fewer side effects. When additional sedation is required, a combination of the antipsychotic medication and an anti-anxiety medication such as lorazepam (Ativan) is safe, effective, and more comfortable for the patient than administering a high dose of the antipsychotic medication.

   Traditionally, it has been said that with very agitated clients one of the more sedating phenothiazines (e.g., Thorazine) is preferred, while a paranoid client who is likely to be very sensitive to "being drugged" might respond better to one of the less sedating medications like Haldol or Prolixin. I prefer to use high-potency, less sedating medications in almost all cases. The high-potency antipsychotics are preferable with very agitated clients because it is possible to safely and rapidly administer a much larger equivalent dose of medication.

There is now active debate about whether clients routinely should be started on one of the newer atypical antipsychotic medications rather than a traditional antipsychotic. Clozapine is too dangerous to use as a first-line drug, but it can be effective for people who have not responded well to other medications. Risperidone, olanzapine, and quetiapine (and the other new atypical medications about to be released) seem safe, well-tolerated, and have fewer side effects than older medications. They are also much more expensive than the older medications. Despite the expense, I now recommend starting new patients on one of the newer medications. Of course, clients should be switched to one of the new atypical antipsychotic medications if they are having problems with a traditional antipsychotic or are experiencing less than a full response.

2. *Schizophrenia.* Symptoms of schizophrenia have been divided into positive symptoms (hallucinations and delusions), negative symptoms (apathy, social withdrawal, loss of spontaneity, lack of pleasure in things), and disorganized symptoms (disorganized thinking and speech). While positive symptoms are more dramatic and more clearly associated with "being crazy," negative symptoms cause more disability and are more associated with poor quality of life. Traditional antipsychotic medications are generally very effective for positive and disorganized symptoms but less effective for negative symptoms. The new atypical antipsychotic medications seem to work on positive, negative, and disorganized symptoms.

   Initial treatment for schizophrenia is targeted on symptom control and helping the person reestablish control over his or her behavior. This might mean helping the person become stable enough to leave the hospital or recover from a crisis.

Often medications are used in somewhat higher doses to help the person get through this period as rapidly as possible. There is no evidence that a high dose of medication works better or faster than a lower dose, but it is important to give enough medication to be effective. When the effective dose for a particular person is unknown, erring a bit high is usually considered better than erring too low. The balance between the need for speed and the risk of uncomfortable side effects must always be considered.

Maintenance treatment must continue to ensure stability, but long-term quality of life issues become the main focus. The majority of clients with schizophrenia will have a relapse if they discontinue their antipsychotic medication. Generally, people with schizophrenia need to be on maintenance antipsychotic medication for many years. Recently, there has been increasing interest in decreasing the client's long-term exposure to medication. Current research suggests that many clients—even those with severe long-term illness—do well with much lower doses of antipsychotic medication, especially if they are monitored closely and given additional medication during periods of relapse. Haloperidol at 5 mg/day or risperidone at 4 mg/day seems as effective as higher doses for most clients with schizophrenia, at least those with fairly recent onset of the illness, and causes many fewer side effects. Attempts have also been made to use a targeted medication strategy where the person does not stay on medication but restarts medication rapidly at the first early sign of a relapse. For most people with schizophrenia, targeted medication strategies lead to more relapses, more rehospitalizations and poorer functioning. For the few patients who do well for periods off medication and who are willing to go back on medication when necessary, this limited use of medication during periods of relapse is possible.

Most clients with schizophrenia do not relapse immediately if they discontinue antipsychotic medication. Research has suggested that a client with schizophrenia who discontinues medication has around a 10% chance of relapsing during the first month. Of those clients who do not relapse during the first month off medication, approximately 10% will relapse in the second month, and so on, with around 10% of the remaining clients relapsing every month they are off medication. Some clients will go many months before relapsing, but this brief period of stability does not mean that medication is no longer needed.

3. *Manic depression—manic phase acute.* Use antipsychotics in a moderate to large dose (e.g., fluphenazine or haloperidol at 5 mg once or twice a day) to control a client until the lithium has had time to become more effective. When more sedation and behavioral control are needed, I combine the antipsychotic with a long-acting benzodiazepine (clonazepam or diazepam) rather than increasing the dose of the antipsychotic. This often allows for behavioral control with fewer side effects. It was once believed that antipsychotic medications were the most effective way to rapidly control the behavior of manic clients. Now, benzodiazepines are being used more frequently to establish behavioral control in hypomanic clients who are not psychotic.

   Recent data suggest that clozapine may be effective in the long-term treatment of manic-depressive disorder that does not respond to more traditional (and safer) mood-stabilizing medications.

4. *Organic brain syndrome (OBS).* Antipsychotic medication is often beneficial in very low doses (Haldol 0.5 to 2 mg hs [before bed] or risperidone 1 mg). Doses should be kept low, as higher doses can cause confusion and behavioral problems to worsen, especially in elderly clients and clients with dementia. Antipsychotic medication can help control both problematic behavior and emotional lability in some OBS clients. Medications should be used only after the medical work-up of the OBS is completed and the diagnosis is firmly established.

5. *Delusional depression.* Clients who are psychotic or suffer delusional depression initially respond much better to the combination of antipsychotic and antidepressant medications than to antidepressants alone. Once the client has begun to respond, the antipsychotic medication can be tapered and then discontinued, leaving the antidepressant for maintenance therapy. Except in very rare cases, antipsychotic medications should not be used as maintenance medication for clients who have previously had a psychotic depression but who are not currently psychotic. Also, some very agitated depressed clients will have a faster feeling of relief and faster agitation reduction if low-dose antipsychotic medications are initially used along with the antidepressants. Again, these medications should be used only for short periods of time in these depressed clients.

   Non-agitated, non-delusional depressed clients are often made worse by antipsychotic medications.Too high a dose of antipsychotic medication can trigger depression in any client.

A Word about Cigarette Smoking and Antipsychotics

Cigarettes induce (increase the activity) of the enzymes that break down antipsychotic (and many other) medications. This means that smokers generally need a higher dose of medication than nonsmokers. It also means that if someone *stops* smoking, his serum level of medication will increase and he may develop medication side effects.

Specifics of Use of Traditional Antipsychotic Medications

1. *Chlorpromazine (Thorazine).* A typical dose range for psychotic clients is 400–1500 mg/day in divided doses. It is commonly said that 400 mg/day is a minimal antipsychotic dose for schizophrenic clients, although there is increasing interest in studying the effectiveness of very low doses. There is little research supporting the use of more than 600–700 mg/day.

Typical prn orders for agitated psychotic clients will be 100 mg PO or 50 mg IM.

This is the most sedating of the traditional antipsychotic medications, which means it is good for some agitated clients but will also have the most sedating side effects. Because it causes clients to feel "drugged" or "zombie like," I rarely prescribe it for use during the day, but it is useful to some clients before sleep.

Chlorpromazine occasionally causes extreme sensitivity to sunlight and can cause opacities in the lens of the eye. The most sedating antipsychotics, such as Thorazine and Mellaril (and clozapine, which is discussed below), also have the most anticholinergic side effects, including dry mouth, blurred vision, constipation, and occasionally urinary retention. These also have the highest frequency of orthostatic hypotension (an abrupt drop in blood pressure when the client stands up).

At the same time, chlorpromazine and thioridazine are much less likely to cause extrapyramidal effects and therefore there is less need to use antiparkinsonian medications to control them.

2. *Thioridazine (Mellaril).* This dose is roughly equivalent to chlorpromazine, except that it should never be used above 800 mg/day and only rarely above 400 mg/day because of its potential to damage the retina, causing blindness. Some experts suggest that caution should be taken when using thioridazine in combination with antidepressant medications (although this is done frequently) because of the risk of heart arrhythmias and sudden death.

   Thioridazine is a sedating medication that seems to be tolerated better than chlorpromazine and has fewer depressant side effects. It does not come in an injectable form and cannot be used in large doses, but it may be useful with a well-controlled client or as a nighttime medication.

   Some research has suggested that Mellaril causes tardive dyskinesia less often than other antipsychotic medications, but this has been hotly debated and remains a controversial subject. The findings have, however, encouraged some physicians to prescribe Mellaril in situations where its restricted dose range and tendency to cause sedation are not problems.

This medication (as well as the other antipsychotics) is also useful for agitated or psychotic depression (200–400 mg/day) and for organic brain syndrome (low doses, i.e., 25 mg hs [before sleep] or bid [twice a day]).

3. *Fluphenazine (Prolixin).* Traditional dose range is 2–40 mg/day, although recent data suggest that the lower end of the range should be used in most cases. This medication is roughly 50 times as potent as chlorpromazine, and is a high-potency, low-dose, "least-sedating" phenothiazine. It can be given by mouth (po) or by short-acting injection (Prolixin hydrochloride), or as a long-acting esterified injectable form that lasts for over 2 weeks called fluphenazine decanoate (Prolixin Decanoate).

4. *Haloperidol (Haldol).* The dose range is 1–40 mg/day, although current research suggests that 5 mg/day is an effective dose for many people with schizophrenia. Haloperidol is chemically a butyrophenone rather than a phenothiazine. Despite this difference in its chemistry, it seems to work identically to the other phenothiazine medications. It is a very high-potency antipsychotic, and like Prolixin, it is roughly 50 times as potent as chlorpromazine. Twenty mg/day of haloperidol is roughly equivalent to 1000 mg chlorpromazine. It also comes in a long-acting injection called haloperidol decanoate (Haldol Decanoate) that can be given once a month.

5. *Thiothixene (Navane).* The dosage is 5–60 mg/day. Thiothixene is roughly 25 times as potent as chlorpromazine. It is chemically similar to chlorpromazine but is only moderately sedating and is advertised as being well-tolerated and having few side effects.

6. *Molindone (Moban).* The dosage is 20–225 mg/day. In most

ways, molindone is very similar to the phenothiazines, except that it may cause less weight gain than do the other antipsychotics. As with Mellaril, some very speculative research suggests that molindone may cause tardive dyskinesia less often than some of the other medications. It is commonly used as a backup for clients who have not responded well to other medications.

Long-Acting Injections

Long-acting injections are particularly useful for clients who might not take their medications after leaving the hospital or when oral medications are not being absorbed. Also, some clients prefer receiving an injection every 2–4 weeks to taking a pill daily. Both fluphenazine (Prolixin) and haloperidol (Haldol) are now available in the United States in a long-acting, injectable preparation. A client who requires the Prolixin or Haldol Decanoate injections after discharge should probably be started on the short-acting form of the same medications as soon as possible so that side effects can be assessed.

Dose equivalency between oral medication and long-acting injection is highly variable from client to client. As a rough rule of thumb, 10 mg/day of oral Prolixin is equivalent to a 12.5 mg (1/2 cc) injection of Prolixin Decanoate every 2 weeks. Ten mg/day of oral Haldol is roughly equivalent to a 100 mg injection of Haldol Decanoate every 4 weeks (i.e., 10 times the daily oral dose, given by injection every month). There is some difference between the two medications' pharmacokinetic properties (the way drugs are absorbed and metabolized or, in other words, the speed of onset and how long they remain in the body). With Prolixin Decanoate, the client tends to establish an effective serum level of medication within a day or two. With Haldol Decanoate, there is a gradual, smoother uptake of medication, and it may take several weeks or more to get an effective serum level. Because of this slow uptake, it is often useful to start Haldol Decanoate with a higher "loading dose" by giving more medication during the first two months and then decreasing to a baseline dose. A patient on 10 mg/day of oral Haldol could be given 200 mg of Haldol Decanoate through several injections during the first two months, and then given slowly decreasing amounts until a baseline dose of 100 mg/month was reached. Prolixin has the advantage of working faster after a single injection but has the disadvantage of having more side effects a few days after each injection.

Haldol Decanoate stays in the body longer than the Prolixin. Haldol Decanoate's half-life is approximately 21 days, which means that it would take five times that, or more than 100 days, for any dose change to completely equilibrate at a new blood level. Most people do well with a Haldol Decanoate injection once a month. Prolixin Decanoate's half-life is approximately 14 days, which means that injections are typically given every two weeks and that it would take 40-60 days for any dose change to equilibrate at a new blood level.

Atypical Antipsychotic Medications

Clozapine was the first "atypical" antipsychotic medication released. Three other atypical antipsychotic medications (risperidone, olanzapine, and now quetiapine) are now available, and it is expected that several others will be available over the next couple of years. These "atypical" antipsychotic medications have a mechanism of action different from traditional neuroleptics. They cause far fewer and far less severe extrapyramidal (muscle) side effects. Clozapine (and probably the other atypical medications) seem much less likely to cause tardive dyskinesia. It has even been suggested that clozapine might make already existing tardive dyskinesia better.

Clozapine seems to be effective in a significant number of people with schizophrenia who have not responded to other antipsychotic medications. Clozapine is also an extremely effective mood stabilizer and can be used to treat bipolar disorders that have not responded to mood stabilizers. The other atypical antipsychotic medications do not seem as effective as Clozapine for patients who have not responded to traditional medications. Finally, the atypical antipsychotic medications seem much more effective with the negative symptoms of schizophrenia than traditional medications.

Clozapine is the most effective antipsychotic now available. It has too many side effects to be a first-line drug, but no client with schizophrenia should be considered unresponsive to medication without being offered a clozapine trail.

---

1. *Clozapine (Clozaril)* is a very sedating medication, has strong anticholinergic side effects (dry mouth, blurred vision, constipation), and causes orthostatic blood pressure drops. Other side effects include fever, headache, nausea, rapid pulse, and increased salivation. It can also cause significant weight gain in some clients. While these side effects can be uncomfortable, they are not usually dangerous. Especially in higher doses, clozapine causes seizures much more frequently than the other antipsychotic medications. There also seems to be a significant risk of heat stroke when clozapine is taken by people exposed to high environmental temperatures.

   Most seriously, 1% of people taking clozapine will develop agranulocytosis (they will stop making white blood cells). If this is discovered in time and the medication is stopped, the client can recover without difficulty. If this drop in white blood cells is not discovered, the person can die from infections that he or she can no longer fight. There were at least thirteen reported deaths from clozapine between 1990 and 1996, even with regular blood testing. Most cases of agranulocytosis occur 6–18 weeks after starting clozapine.

   Currently, anyone taking clozapine is required to get a weekly count of white blood cells to ensure that they are still being made. More frequent monitoring is required for people who have mild decreases in the total white cell count to 3,000–3,500. Anyone with a total white count below 3,000 or a granulocyte count (mature white cell count) of less than 1,500 must immediately discontinue clozapine. Currently, in the United States, a client can get medication only a week at a time and cannot receive the next week's medication without first obtaining a blood test. Unfortunately, this means that clients who do not want to put up with the hassle of weekly tests cannot benefit from the medication. It also means that clozapine can be prescribed only when an organized monitoring system is in place.

It is expected that the U.S. Food and Drug Administration (FDA) soon will allow people who have been taking clozapine for more than six months to decrease the frequency of these blood counts. This may expose clients to slight additional risk, but many clients would prefer this risk to the weekly blood tests.

This monitoring system makes clozapine extremely expensive. Medical assistance programs in many states require prior authorization for clozapine, which is not required for any other medication. For clients who have neither medical assistance nor insurance, the cost of the medication can preclude its use.

To decrease the risk of seizures and other side effects, clozapine is usually started at 12.5 or 25 mg/day and then increased by 25 mg every 3 days until a dose of 300–450 mg is reached by the end of 2–3 weeks. Subsequent increases should be no more than 25 mg at a time, with increases no more frequent than twice a week. The majority of clients respond to 300–600 mg/day. The maximum dose is 900 mg/day, but seizures are more frequent above 600 mg. It is now suggested that anyone taking clozapine in high doses also take divalproex sodium (Depakote) to decrease the risk of seizures. Depakote is commonly used in psychiatry as a mood stabilizer (discussed later), but its primary use in medicine is as an anticonvulsant. It is recommended that clozapine be taken twice a day, but in the lower end of the dose range it seems safe and effective to give it once a day if side effects are carefully monitored. There are some data suggesting that clozapine is more effective if the serum level is above 350 ng/ml.

Clozapine may take a long time to be effective. Some clients who do not respond after 4 weeks at a full dose will show a later response, and many clients who intially have only a partial response will respond better after taking the medication for 6 months or more.

Drug-Drug Interactions. There is potential risk in combining clozapine with a benzodiazepine, especially if the dose is rapidly increased. This combination has resulted in at least seven reported incidents of people stopping breathing. Given the number of patients who have had no problems taking clozapine and a benzodiazepine, the risk of stopping breathing appears very low. Confusion, sedation, and increased salivation from the combination have also been reported.

Caffeine is reported to increase clozapine levels in some patients, while smoking can lower them. SSRI-type antidepressants can increase clozapine levels, and anticonvulsants, including valproate, can decrease them. Medications used outside of psychiatry can also affect clozapine levels. For example, the antibiotic erythromycin and the antiulcer medication cimetidine can increase clozapine levels to potentially dangerous levels.

2. *Risperidone (Risperdal)* was the second new-generation atypical antipsychotic medication to be marketed. When used in the recommended dose range of 4–6 mg/day, it has few extrapyramidal side effects, which gives it a major advantage over older medications. Some data indicate that it may be effective in clients who have not responded to other medications, and it seems more effective in decreasing negative symptoms. Risperidone may also have some antidepressant activity.

The main advantage of risperidone is that it has few side effects. Weight gain is a commonly reported problem, although it is less problematic with risperidone than with clozapine. Risperidone commonly causes elevation of prolactin, a hormone that can cause various sexual side effects, including amenorrhea in women. Orthostatic hypotension (sudden drops in blood pressure when the client stands quickly) may be a problem and may require that the medication be divided and given twice a day. Insomnia and agitation are more often reported rather than the sedation seen with most other antipsychotic medications. Akathisia is also sometimes reported but is less frequent and less severe than with the traditional antipsychotic medications. Other side effects are rare if the dose does not go above 6 mg/day. Potential side effects include akathisia, anxiety, runny nose, and nausea. Sexual side effects may occur along with prolactin elevations. Any medication can cause agranulocytosis, but the incidence of this with risperidone appears to be very low and no special blood tests or monitoring are required. The incidence of seizures also seems very low.

A full dose of risperidone for most people with schizophrenia is 4–6 mg/day. Two mg/day seems less effective, at least for most clients with schizophrenia, and increasing the dose to more than 6 mg/day can cause a significant increase in extrapyramidal side effects with no apparent increase in effectiveness. Risperidone has a half-life of around 20 hours, which means that most people can take it once a day without problems.

In elderly demented clients, very small amounts of risperidone (0.5–1 mg/day) are often useful in controlling psychotic symptoms and agitation. It has begun to replace haloperidol as the preferred antipsychotic for these clients.

Risperidone is an expensive medication. A standard dose of 6 mg/day costs over $2,800 per year.

3. *Olanzapine (Zyprexa)* is one of the newest atypical antipsychotics to be marketed in the United States. It seems effective

and very well tolerated. It has a very low incidence of motor side effects when used below 20 mg/day, and, like risperidone, it seems to have an extremely low incidence of blood dyscrasias or seizures. Common side effects include drowsiness, dizziness, dry mouth, and orthostatic blood pressure drops. Weight gain is a common problem, as with all of the atypical antipsychotic medications. Olanzapine causes significantly more weight gain than risperidone but less than clozapine. Agitation, nausea, and indigestion are rarer but have also been reported. Olanzapine does not cause the elevation of prolactin seen in traditional antipsychotic medications and seems to have fewer sexual side effects than older medications. Increases in liver enzymes have been reported but are not considered a problem until they are twice the normal values.

A typical dose of olanzapine is 10–20 mg/day. In a healthy adult, 10 mg can be given as the starting dose, although there will be less initial sedation if 5 mg is used first and then increased after a day or two. EPSE (motor) side effects, especially akathisia, become more common in doses above 20 mg/day. Olanzapine may also have some mood-stabilizing properties.

4. *Quetiapine (Seroquel)* was released in October 1997. It seems both effective and well tolerated. It has essentially no extrapyramidal side effects and fairly low anticholinergic side effects. It also causes no prolactin elevation, which suggests that it might have fewer sexual side effects than some of the other antipsychotic medications. It is slightly more sedating than olanzapine, but much less sedating than clozapine. It causes a slight increase in pulse and a temporary release of enzymes from the liver into the blood. This increase in circulating liver enzymes is reported as an abnormality in some tests of liver function. These effects are seldom problematic. Orthostatic hypotension (temporary drop in blood pressure when standing suddenly) is a problem for some clients. Weight gain may also be a problem for some clients taking quetiapine, as it is for all the atypical antipsychotics.

Quetiapine has a short half-life of 6 hours, which suggests it might need to be taken twice a day by at least some clients. It is usually started at 25 mg twice a day, with a typical range of 300–400mg/day and a maximum dose of 750 mg/day.

5. *Ziprasidone (Zeldox)* is expected to be marketed soon. It is a short-acting medication that will need to be taken twice a day. It is the first activating antipsychotic medication. While it may cause some sedation when first started, agitation and insomnia are much more common. Early reports suggest that combining ziprasidone with lorazepam, especially when starting treatment, can decrease the agitation and insomnia. Initial reports suggest that it causes fewer side effects than other antipsychotics, including fewer sexual side effects and less weight gain.

Side Effects

Side effects of the antipsychotic medications can be divided into three broad categories. The first is extrapyramidal, or muscle-related, side effects. The second group includes common, non-muscle-related side effects that are uncomfortable but not life-threatening, and the third covers those that are rare, dangerous, and can lead to permanent difficulties.

Extrapyramidal Effects

Pyramidal cells are nerve cells in the brain that are involved in the control of voluntary muscle movements. Extrapyramidal refers to the part of the central nervous system concerned with control and coordination of muscle movements not part of the main pyramidal tracts (hence the term extrapyramidal). These are common and uncomfortable but not dangerous complications of antipsychotic drug use. They can increase the discomfort of many clients and frequently prompt clients to refuse to take medications. They are usually treatable, and, except for tardive dyskinesia, all disappear when drugs are discontinued. Tardive dyskinesia has no reliable treatment and may be permanent even after antipsychotic medications are stopped.

Extrapyramidal side effects are much less frequent with the new atypical antipsychotic medications, including clozapine, risperidone, and olanzapine. In addition, the atypical antipsychotic medications appear less likely to cause tardive dyskinesia.

1. *Dystonia* symptoms include sudden, often dramatic, spasms of muscles of head, neck, lips, and tongue. Tilted head, slurred speech, or eyes deviated up or to one side are also common. Dystonias can be very frightening and at times are dismissed as bizarre behavior rather than recognized as a drug side effect. Dystonias usually occur hours or days after the medication is started or the dose is increased. They are easily treated with anticholinergic drugs like benztropine (Cogentin) 1–2 mg po or IM, or diphenhydramine (Benadryl) 25 mg IM for rapid relief.

2. *Pseudoparkinsonism* usually consists of muscular rigidity, mask-like face, and stiff walk with loss of normal arm swing and a shuffling gait. These clients often have a coarse, 3 per/sec tremor that is worse at rest than with activity. Pseudoparkinsonism usually begins after 3 weeks of treatment.

3. *Akathisia* is a late appearing side effect that usually occurs 5–14 days after beginning medication. It is characterized by constant pacing, moving of hands or feet, and a feeling of nervousness. Clients can often distinguish this motor restlessness from anxiety and may say things like "it feels like my motor is running all of the time."

Akathisia is a common, very uncomfortable, and often unrecognized side effect that is one of the frequent reasons that clients discontinue their medication.

Akathisia often becomes more severe if the person is already anxious and can become somewhat better if the person can relax. This can be very confusing since akathisia is easily confused with anxiety in the first place. Akathisia can also be confused with an exacerbation of the underlying psychosis. Some clients find that caffeine makes it worse. Beta-blockers such as propranolol, benzodiazepines such as clonazepam, anticholinergic medications such as benztropine (Cogentin), and reducing the dose of the antipsychotic medication can all be useful, but uncomfortable symptoms may persist.

4. *Akinesia* is frequently overlooked and can be difficult to distinguish from the psychiatric illness for which the drug is being prescribed. It is manifested by loss of spontaneity in facial expression or gesturing, being "slowed up," or shuffling. More subtle but still uncomfortable parts of this syndrome are seen in decreased social spontaneity, diminished conversation, apathy and disinclination to initiate normal activity. Akinesia is partially treatable with anticholinergic medication, but it is often treatment resistant and can be an ongoing clinical problem.

5. *Tardive dyskinesia* appears late, usually after years of medication use, and seems to be related to total lifetime dose of medication. Once it appears in full-blown syndrome, *it can be permanent*. It is estimated to affect 20–30% of clients chronically using antipsychotic medications and appears more frequently in women, older clients, and clients having a diagnosis other than schizophrenia. It can be stopped by early recognition and discontinuation of the antipsychotic medication. Some studies have suggested that abnormally frequent eye-blinking may be an early sign of tardive dyskinesia in some clients. In other clients, the first sign is a writhing motion of the tongue. If the medication is continued, this can progress to rhythmic, disfiguring distortion of the mouth or face. Other parts of the body can also be involved. There are a number of common scales, including the AIMS (abnormal involuntary movement scale), that allow clinicians to monitor and track early symptoms of tardive dyskinesia.

   Some clients who get very mild tardive dyskinesia find that it never worsens, even if they stay on antipsychotic medications. In other clients it can progress fairly rapidly over a period of months to become a very disfiguring and incapacitating movement disorder. It is impossible to predict who is at risk for progression to the severe form and who is not. As more clients are treated with antipsychotic agents for longer periods of time, tardive dyskinesia is likely to become increasingly problematic.

Cogentin and other anticholinergic drugs can usually control most extrapyramidal side effects, but they often make tardive dyskinesia worse rather than better. As with other extrapyramidal side effects, symptoms of tardive dyskinesia typically disappear with sleep and are made worse by increased anxiety. Similarly, caffeine often makes symptoms worse, although this varies from one client to another. There is some suggestion that vitamin E may decrease the chance of developing tardive dyskinesia and may be partially helpful in its treatment.

Common, Uncomfortable, But Usually Temporary or Reversible Side Effects

6. *Toxic side effects* generally affect everyone taking antipsychotic medications, at least to some extent. They are usually dose-related and sometimes can be controlled by changing doses, taking most of the dose at night, or switching medications. They include drowsiness, feeling "drugged," sluggish, and unmotivated. They are often worse with Thorazine than with the high-potency antipsychotics. Clients become partially tolerant to these symptoms over time. Drug-induced or drug-potentiated depressions also may occur.

7. *Psychotoxic effects* include depression, depersonalization, dysphoria, akinesia, confusion, and somatic delusion. *Remember, antipsychotic drugs can makes things worse as well as better.* These side effects, which are connected to the feeling of being "drugged," all seem to be much less of a problem with the new atypical antipsychotic medications.

8. *Autonomic side effects.* Autonomic side effects refer to the effects on what is called the involuntary or vegetative nervous system. This is the part of the nervous system responsible for maintaining basic processes in the body, such as temperature regulation and blood pressure. This system involves two neurotransmitters, acetylcholine and epinephrine. All of these medications block the action of acetylcholine to a greater or lesser extent, and therefore cause all of the side effects of other anticholinergic drugs (discussed below). The most common anticholinergic side effects include dry mouth, blurred vision, and constipation. These medications also block some of the actions of epinephrine, causing other autonomic side effects such as orthostatic hypotension (sudden drop in blood pressure when the client suddenly stands up), which can cause some transient dizziness and, in extreme cases, can cause the client to fall down. All of these side effects are worse with low-potency drugs like Thorazine and Mellaril and are a particular problem with clozapine.

9. *Endocrine effects.* Weight gain is a problem with any antipsychotic medication. Not all people taking these medications gain weight, but the medications clearly make it more likely. Weight gain seems worse with clozapine and the other new atypical antipsychotic medications. There is supposedly less weight gain with molindone (Moban).

   All the traditional antipsychotic medications and some of the atypicals (e.g., risperidone) increase prolactin, one of the sexual-related hormones. Prolactin elevation can interfere with menstruation and can cause lactation (even in men).

10. *Sexual dysfunction.* Both men and women describe decreased sexual desire. In addition, these medications can cause problems with erection in men. Mellaril can also cause retrograde ejaculation (erection and ejaculation are normal but semen is pushed backward into the bladder instead of the penis).

11. *Skin reactions* include rashes, itching, and some swelling.

Symptoms usually begin 1–5 weeks after beginning treatment. Thorazine is the most common offender. These rashes are uncomfortable but usually are not dangerous.

12. *Photosensitivity reactions.* Skin can become very sensitive to sunlight. Again, Thorazine is the most common drug involved.

Rare but Serious and Potentially Permanent Side Effects

13. *Blood dyscrasias.* Many clients put on these drugs have a partial block on production of certain blood elements, usually white cells and platelets. This is usually of no clinical significance and within a few days the system is back to normal. Occasionally the white blood count continues to decrease slowly (leukopenia) in a dose-related reaction without other symptoms. This decrease must be monitored closely, and sometimes switching to a different medication is necessary. If this temporary block is relatively complete and the system does not return to normal, the rapid decrease in white cells and/or platelets quickly becomes life-threatening. Such a complete block is very rare but is relatively more common with low-potency, high-dose drugs (Thorazine and Mellaril). It is *much* more common with clozapine (Clozaril).

People are at highest risk for a block in making white blood cells (agranulocytosis) in the first two to four months after starting a new medication.

The block on production of white blood cells is more common in debilitated clients. Symptoms include weakness, high fever, chills, and a sore throat. A physician should be called and a CBC (complete blood count) ordered immediately. The outcome depends on how rapidly diagnosis is made. If the client has a blood dyscrasia, all medication must be stopped immediately.

14. *Neuroleptic malignant syndrome (NMS)* usually occurs within a few weeks of starting an antipsychotic medication and is marked by a very high temperature and muscle stiffness.

Clients can easily die from hyperthermia (temperature above 105°) if not rapidly and vigorously treated.

Any client taking an antipsychotic medication who complains of an increased temperature and muscular rigidity should be evaluated for NMS.

Other early signs include confusion, increased pulse, and increased blood pressure.

15. *Temperature regulation.* All antipsychotic medications can interfere with a person's normal temperature-regulation mechanisms in hot weather. During the 1995 heat wave a number of people taking these medications died, including several young men who would not normally be considered at risk for fatal heat stroke.

Clients on antipsychotic medications, especially low-potency medications such as clozapine and chlorpromazine (Thorazine), are much more likely to suffer a potentially fatal heatstroke.

Clients taking these medications should have air conditioners or fans, or have a cool place to go if their living accommodations become too hot. They should also drink fluids to avoid becoming dehydrated.

16. *Cardiovascular effects.* Many medications slightly increase the time it takes for electrical impulses to spread through the heart. They also increase the time required for the heart to "repolarize," or reset, after the last heartbeat in preparation for the next beat. Very occasionally, these medications will cause the heart to beat irregularly, especially when they are combined with other medications that have a similar effect on the heart or when given to people with certain kinds of heart disease. Mellaril seems to cause arrhythmias more often than the other medications. It should be used with caution in people diagnosed as having problems with normal conduction of electrical impulses through the heart. Sudden death from irregular heartbeat has been reported as a very rare side effect of all of these drugs.

17. *Eye problems.* Blurred vision is a common, reversible side effect from all of these medications, especially the high-dose medications like Thorazine and Mellaril. This is an "anticholinergic" side effect and is made worse by other anticholinergic medications, including medications used for extrapyramidal side effects such as Cogentin or by antidepressants such as Elavil. The blurred vision goes away when the medication is discontinued.

    Lens opacities (cataracts) are a rare but more serious side effect, especially of long-term Thorazine use. Mellaril has been reported to cause deposition of the pigments in the retina that can lead to blindness. This is extremely rare in clients taking less than 800 mg/day for a lengthy period of time.

18. *Seizures.* All of these medications lower the seizure threshold. Seizures are rare in people taking these medications but are something to consider, especially with clients who already have difficultly controlling epilepsy. Some of these medications, such as clozapine, are much more likely to cause seizures than other antipsychotic medications, especially when used in higher doses. Seizures are rarely dangerous (unless the person happens to be driving at the time), but they are frightening to both the client and observers.

Use during Pregnancy

It cannot be proven that any medication is absolutely safe during pregnancy. These drugs do cross the placenta, but there is no evidence that antipsychotic medications increase the risk of birth defects. While all pregnant women should, as a general rule, take as few medications as possible, pregnancy should not be a reason to completely avoid antipsychotic drug use. The stress of psychosis is also potentially damaging to the fetus, and the various risks must be weighed against each other. These drugs will also appear in breast milk. Again, while there is no absolute contraindication, it is probably safer for mothers taking these medications not to breast feed their babies.

TABLE 4. *Side Effects and Potency of Antipsychotic Medications*

	Doses equivalent to 100 mg of chlorpromazine	Sedation	Anticholinergic side effects	EPSE	Orthostatic hypotension
chlorpromazine (Thorazine)	100 mg	+ + +	+ +	+ +	+ + +
clozapine (Clozaril)	50 mg	+ + +	+ + +	+ /0	+ + +
fluphenazine (Prolixin)	2 mg	+	+	+ + +	+
haloperidol (Haldol)	2 mg	+	+	+ + +	+
loxapine (Loxitane)	10 mg	+ +	+	+ + +	+ +
mesoridazine (Serentil)	50 mg	+ + +	+ + +	+	+ +
molindone (Moban)	10 mg	+	+	+ + +	+
olanzapine (Zyprexa)	5 mg	+ +	+	+ /0	+
perphenazine (Trilafon)	8 mg	+	+	+ + +	+
prochlorperazine (Compazine)	15 mg	+ +	+	+ + +	+
risperidone (Risperdal)	2 mg	+	+	+	+
thioridazine (Mellaril)	100 mg	+ + +	+ + +	+	+ + +
thiothixene (Navane)	4 mg	+	+	+ + +	+
trifluoperazine (Stelazine)	5 mg	+	+	+ + +	+

Key: + Mild + + Moderate + + + Severe +/0 Minimal

Adapted from *Drug Facts and Comparisons*, 1997, St. Louis, MO: Facts and Comparisons.

TABLE 5. *Most Commonly Reported Side Effects of Atypical Antipsychotic Medications (listed in order of frequency)*

Clozapine	Risperidone	Olanzapine	Quetiapine
Drowsiness	Insomnia	Tiredness	Agitation
Increased salivation	Agitation	Asthenia	Tiredness
Increased pulse	Akasthisia	Dizziness	Headache
Dizziness	Headache	SGPT increase	Dizziness
Constipation	Anxiety	Constipation	Constipation
Orthostatic hypotension	Runny nose	Increased pulse	Dry mouth

Adapted from "Current Psychotropic Dosing and Monitoring Guidelines," by L. Ereshefsky, G. P. Overman, and J. K. Karp, July 1996, *Primary Psychiatry* 3(7), p. 37. Reprinted by permission of *Primary Psychiatry*.

TABLE 6. *Detailed Side Effect Profile of Atypical Antipsychotic Medications*

	typical antipsychotic	clozapine	risperidone	olanzapine	quetiapine	ziprasidone
Agitation	+ to + +	0	+/-	+	+	0
Agranulocytosis	rare	+ + +	rare	rare	rare	rare
Anticholinergic	+ to +++	+ + +	+/-	+ +	+ +	+
Liver enzyme abnormalities	+	+	0	+	+	+
EPSE	+ to + + +	0	+	0	0	+
Dose-related EPSE increase	yes	no	yes	yes	yes	yes
Nausea/ heartburn	+	0	+/-	+	0	+
Orthostatic hypotension	+ to + + +	+ + +	+ +	+ +	+ +	+ +
Prolactin increase	+ to + +	0	+ +	+	0	+
Sedation	+ + to + + +	+ + +	+ +	+	0	+
Seizures	+	+ + + dose-related	+	+	+	+
Tardive dyskinesia	+ + +	0	?	?	?	?
Weight gain	+	+ + +	+ +	+ +	+ +	?

KEY: + Mild + + Moderate + + + Severe +/- Minimal ? Uncertain 0 None

From "A Summary of Research Findings on New Antipsychotic Drugs," by M. D. Jibson and R. Tandon, May 1996, *The Psychiatry Forum*, 16, p. iv.

TABLE 7. *Common Side Effects of Medications Used to Treat Schizophrenia*

Side Effect	Description	May be confused with ...
Akasthisia	• Feeling restless or jittery • Needing to fidget, stand up, or pace around	• Anxiety • Psychotic symptoms • Cocaine intoxication • Alcohol withdrawal
Akinesia	• Feeling slowed-down • Losing normal spontaneity • No mental energy ("I feel like a zombie")	• Negative symptoms of schizophrenia • Depression
Anticholinergic side effects (physical)	• Dry mouth • Blurry vision • Trouble urinating • Constipation	none
Anticholinergic side effects (mental effects)	• Memory difficulties • Confusion (feeling "spacy") • Visual hallucinations	• Symptoms of schizophrenia • Drug intoxication • Depression
Dystonia	• Sudden muscle spasm; charleyhorse (usually happens when antipsychotic medication is started or dose raised; most common with high-potency traditional antipsychotics)	• Strange movements that occur during psychotic episodes • Dystonia may be triggered by stress and may be mistaken for hysterical reactions or malingering
Sexual and menstrual difficulties	• Loss of sexual desire • Loss of erection or ejaculation • Cessation of menses	• Low sex drive can also be due to schizophrenia or depression • Menstrual irregularities
often		caused by medications, and
	rarely directly caused by	schizophrenia
Tardive dyskinesia	• Writhing movements of mouth, tongue, or hands	• Tremor • Transient movements associated with antipsychotic dose reductions • Spontaneous movements seen in people with schizophrenia even without medication exposure
Tremor	• Shaking of hands or other parts of body	
Weight gain	• Common with all antipsychotics, but usually worse with atypical antipsychotics	• Also associated with inactivity and poor diet

Adapted with permission from "The Expert Consensus Guideline Series: Treatment of Schizophrenia," by J. P. McEvoy, P. J. Weiden, T. E. Smith et al., 1996, *Journal of Clinical Psychiatry*, 1996:57 (supplement 12B), p. 55. Copyright 1996 by Expert Knowledge Systems, LLC.

TABLE 8. *Side Effects from Receptor Blockade*

Blockade of dopamine D2 receptors

- Extrapyramidal (muscle) effects: dystonia, tremor, akathisia, tardive dyskinesia, rabbit syndrome
- Endocrine effects: prolactin elevation (galactorrhea, gynecomastia, menstrual changes, sexual dysfunction)

Blockade of acetylcholine (muscarinic) receptors

- Blurred vision, exacerbation of narrow angle glaucoma, dry mouth, increased pulse, constipation, urinary retention, memory dysfunction

Blockade of histamine H1 receptors

- Drowsiness, weight gain

Blockade of alpha1 adrenergic receptors

- Orthostatic hypotension, dizziness.

Adapted from "Preclinical Pharmacology of Neuroleptics: Focus on New Generation Compounds," by E. Richelson, 1996, *Journal of Clinical Psychiatry*, 57(11), p. 8.

4

Antiparkinsonian Medications

Some of the medications commonly used for Parkinson's disease are also useful in treating the Parkinsonian-like, muscle-related side effects of the antipsychotic medications. As was already discussed, the less-sedating antipsychotic medications are more apt to cause these extrapyramidal, muscle-related side effects (EPSE). These include dystonias (muscle spasms), tremors, akasthisia (motor restlessness), and akinesia (decreased spontaneity of movements and thought). The new atypical antipsychotic medications are much less likely to cause extrapyramidal side effects and therefore antiparkinsonian medications are rarely needed.

Some clinicians maintain that it is better to use these medications only after a side effect appears. I generally do not start them when using thioridazine (Mellaril) or chlorpromazine (Thorazine), but on occasion I use them from the beginning when prescribing high-potency antipsychotics like haloperidol (Haldol) or fluphenazine (Prolixin). I am also more likely to start one of these medications at the outset of antipsychotic therapy when I am prescribing larger doses of antipsychotics, when I am treating younger clients (where EPSE seem more common), and when I am treating paranoid clients who are likely to react severely to a side effect.

Antiparkinson (anticholinergic) medications are useful for the muscle-related side effects of antipsychotic medications, but can worsen many other side effects like dry mouth and sedation.

Anticholinergics, e.g., Benztropine (Cogentin)

Specifics of Use

Benztropine (Cogentin) should be taken at 2–8 mg/day in divided doses. Many clients feel that taking the medication once a day is enough, but all antiparkinsonian medications are fairly short-acting and most clients will find that they "wear off" if not taken at least twice a day. I usually start with 1–2 mg twice/day, except with elderly clients, who need lower doses and with whom much more caution should be taken. On prn (use only as needed) orders I usually write for 2 mg IM or po. With severe dystonias or akathisia, the client might be so uncomfortable that intramuscular or intravenous medication is desirable. Other commonly used anticholinergic antiparkinsonian medications include:

- trihexyphenidyl (Artane)—usual dose 2–15 mg/day
- procyclidine (Kemadrin)—usual dose 6–20 mg/day
- biperiden (Akineton)—usual dose 2–8 mg/day

Side Effects

Antiparkinsonian medications are all anticholinergic—that is, they work by blocking the neurotransmitter acetylcholine. As such, they cause the same autonomic side effects as other medications with anticholinergic effects, including most of the antipsychotic medications and many of the antidepressants. These side effects include dry mouth, blurred vision, and constipation. Less frequently, urinary retention, nasal congestion, and muscular weakness become problems. These medications can cause some kinds of glaucoma to worsen or can precipitate glaucoma in people who are already predisposed to develop it. Finally, all these medications can cause memory and other cognitive impairments, especially in elderly clients. It is important to remember that while these medications make some side effects of the antipsychotic medications better, they make other side effects worse.

These medications are nonaddictive but are sometimes abused. They produce a strange kind of "altered state" that some people find enjoyable, and as a result they have street value. In higher doses they produce a delirium where the person becomes disoriented, loses touch with reality, and sometimes becomes delusional or starts hallucinating. This delirium can be confused with psychosis. When a client on one of these or other anticholinergic medications (which include many of the antipsychotics and antidepressants) becomes confused and out of touch with reality, it is important to determine whether the person is psychotic or delirious.

Diphenhydramine (Benadryl)

This is a sedating antihistamine that can also be used as a sedative hypnotic (sleeping pill). It also has strong anticholinergic properties that make it useful for treating medication-induced extrapyramidal side effects. Its anticholinergic effects and mild sedation make it particularly useful for treating akathisia in some clients. Its effects and side effects are very similiar to the other anticholinergic medications.

Amantadine (Symmetrel)

Amantadine has a completely different mechanism of action than the other medications used to treat EPSE. The antipsychotic medications all work by blocking the action of dopamine. This dopamine blockade accounts for the antipsychotics' beneficial effects as well as their extrapyramidal side effects. The anticholinergic medications work by blocking the action of the neurotransmitter acetylcholine. Dopamine and acetylcholine work to balance each other in the part of the brain that controls for extrapyramidal movement. The antipsychotic medications disrupt the balance by blocking dopamine, and the anticholinergics restore the balance by blocking acetylcholine. Amantadine, on the other hand, seems to work by selectively boosting the action of the neurotransmitter dopamine. The best guess about the action of amantadine is that it boosts the action of dopamine in the part of the brain that is associated with extrapyramidal and other side effects and has minimal or no effects on dopamine in the part of the brain associated with the antipsychotic properties of the antipsychotic medications.

Amantadine has no anticholinergic side effects and many clients tolerate it better than other antiparkinsonian medications. Unfortunately, amantadine is less reliable than the anticholinergic medications are, and it may lose its effectiveness over time in some clients. Occasionally clients discontinue amantadine immediately after starting it because they report that it makes them extremely anxious. However, this is unusual and the medication is typically well tolerated. It is now suggested that besides blocking the extrapyramidal side effects of the antipsychotic medications, amantadine may also block other autonomic side effects of the antipsychotics, including weight gain and decreased libido.

The usual dose is 100 mg twice/day, which may be increased to 300 mg/day.

Other Medications Used to Treat Akathisia

Akathisia is very uncomfortable and often very difficult to treat. It is one of the more common reasons that people discontinue antipsychotic medications and has even been cited as a cause of suicide. Akathisia is often unresponsive to anticholinergic medications. Beta-blocking medications such as propranolol (Inderal) are often effective in treating akathisia. Anxiolytics (minor tranquilizers) such as diazepam (Valium) can also be very helpful with akathisia that is unresponsive to other treatment.

Decreasing caffeine use can also decrease akathisia.

5

Antidepressant Medications

There are four main classes of antidepressant medications. They are (1) selective serotonin reuptake inhibitors (SSRIs), such as fluoxetine (Prozac) and sertraline (Zoloft); (2) a heterogeneous group of new-generation medications, such as nefazodone (Serzone) and mirtazapine (Remeron); (3) the tricyclic medications, such as amitriptyline and desipramine; and (4) the monoamine oxidase inhibitors (MAOIs), such as phenelzine (Nardil) and tranylcypromine (Parnate). Medications within any one class are more similar to each other than they are different, and differences within one class are primarily differences in side effects. As with the antipsychotic medications, some clients will respond much better to one medication than to another, even if the medications are similiar and from the same class.

Indications for Use

1. *Depression.* It is often difficult to predict which depressed clients will respond to antidepressant medications and which clients will not. Clients who are more likely to respond to medication may be experiencing weight loss, waking in the early morning, feeling worse in the morning but better as the day goes on, or suffering from depressions lacking a major reactive component (that is, there is no obvious reason why the client is depressed). A pervasive sense of anhedonia (when things the person used to enjoy are no longer fun) and

a sense of hopelessness are other classic characteristics of depressed people who respond to antidepressant medications. Many of these clients have a family member who is depressed, alcoholic, or has made suicide attempts. It may be well worth giving the client a trial of antidepressant medication, even without a clear endogenous pattern, especially if the depression is long-standing and has not responded to psychosocial treatments.

Most clients with a depression do very well with just one antidepressant and do not need a combination of different medications. Clients who are agitated or have a major sleep problems may respond faster if given an antianxiety medication, such as diazepam (Valium), for a few days at the beginning of treatment, in addition to an antidepressant. Some clients with a very agitated depression, especially if they have psychotic symptoms, intially respond better to a combination of an antipsychotic medication and an antidepressant. Clients with a delusional depression initially respond much better to antipsychotic and antidepressant medications than to antidepressants alone. Antidepressant medications seem ineffective in clients going through a typical grief reaction or with a depression that seems primarily reactive to life events.

These medications can be used with antipsychotics, common sleeping pills, or electroconvulsive therapy (ECT). Antidepressants are useful in combination with lithium or other mood stabilizers in clients who are in the depressed phase of a manic-depressive illness.

Always obtain a medication history first. The best antidepressant to start with is one that worked in the past for either that client or someone in his or her immediate family.

2. *Panic Attacks.* These medications are called "antidepressants" because they were first used to treat depression. They are, however, effective for a number of other conditions, and they just as easily could have been called "anti-panic" medications. These medications are not particularly useful for generalized anxiety, but many of the antidepressant medications, with the

exception of bupropion (Wellbutrin), are more effective in decreasing the frequency of true panic attacks than antianxiety medications such as Valium and Librium. Many people with agoraphobia have a combination of panic along and anticipatory anxiety. Antidepressants will often block the panic without affecting the anticipatory anxiety, which is most effectively treated with behavioral therapy.

3. *Obsessive compulsive disorder (OCD).* OCD had until recently been considered unresponsive to medication. An increasing number of research studies have demonstrated that all the SSRIs are extremely helpful with many clients who have this often disabling disorder. OCD often requires a much higher dose of medication than does depression. For example, 20 mg of fluoxetine (Prozac) is generally an effective dose with depressed clients, but people with OCD typically require 60–80 mg/day. Clomipramine (Anafranil) is the most effective medication for OCD, but I do not use it as my first medication of choice because it has many more side effects than the SSRIs. Clomipramine is sedating, causes weight gain, dry mouth, and constipation, and is lethal when taken as an overdose. However, it sometimes helps with OCD when other medications are ineffective. Typically, one starts clomipramine at 25 mg/day and then increases the dose to 150 mg/day. A typical dose range is 150–250 mg/day.

4. *Bulimia.* There are reasonable data indicating that most of the antidepressants (including all of the tricyclics and SSRIs) are useful for at least some people with bulimia, whether they are depressed or not. These medications can decrease the frequency and severity of the bingeing and help people with bulimia to establish more control over their own eating.

5. *Cocaine craving and depression.* It has been proposed that antidepressants may be useful in helping people cope with symptoms of cocaine withdrawal. Desipramine has been most frequently studied, but other antidepressants have also been rumored to be effective for this purpose. Recent data suggest that antidepressants are useful in treating the post-withdraw-

al depression that is very common in heavy, habitual users, but there is much less support for the idea that these medications help with cocaine cravings or withdrawal. As is the case with treating depression, there is often a delay of several weeks between starting the medication and seeing a positive response.

6. *Smoking cessation.* Bupropion, in combination with a nicotine patch and a smoking cessation program, seems effective in helping motivated people quit smoking. This is specific to buproprin. Other antidepressants do not appear effective in decreasing smoking. The bupropion should be started 7-10 days before the designated "stop smoking" day, while the nicotine patch is started when the cigarettes are stopped. Generally, a normal antidepressant dose is used. Bupropion can be started at 100 bid for three days and then increased to 150 bid. Bupropion is marketed under the name Wellbutrin when used as an antidepressant and as Zyban when used as part of a smoking cessation program. They are exactly the same medication.
7. *Miscellaneous.* Antidepressants are also useful for a variety of other conditions. They can increase the effectiveness of some pain medications and are used to treat some migraine-type headaches. They can treat a variety of what are called "stage four sleep disorders," which include night terrors and enuresis in children. Finally, they are effective for some kinds of school avoidance when other therapy has failed.

Selective Serotonin Reuptake Inhibitors (SSRIs)

A number of new antidepressants that block the reuptake of serotonin into nerve cells in the brain have recently been developed. These new antidepressants are extremely selective, blocking only the targeted neurotransmitter, which decreases the number of side effects. SSRIs include fluoxetine (Prozac), sertraline (Zoloft), and paroxetine (Paxil). Prozac was the first of these new antidepressants and was widely publicized as something of a "miracle drug." It was even featured on the cover of *Newsweek*. It has also been attacked by various groups for precipitating suicides, although data do not support this claim. The reality is that these new medications are not miracle drugs, but they are much safer and are generally better tolerated than the older medications.

While these medications do not appear to be any more effective overall than other medications, they may work well for certain clients who do not respond to traditional antidepressants. These serotonergic antidepressants may be particularly useful for clients with both a character disorder and a depression. SSRI antidepressants also seem to be more effective than other antidepressants in treating obsessive compulsive disorder.

Specifics of Use

1. *Fluoxetine (Prozac)*. Most depressed patients respond to a single 20 mg tablet a day, although older clients may not tolerate this high a dose, and most clients with obsessive compulsive disorder require up to 60 mg/day. Fluoxetine has a half-life of more than 80 hours, which means it remains in the body for weeks after someone stops taking it. There are potentially dangerous interactions between serotonergic antidepressants like fluoxetine and a number of other commonly used medications, including other antidepressants, particularly MAOIs. They can dramatically raise the serum level of tricyclic antidepressants and a number of other commonly used medications, including carbamazepine.

   There should be at least a five-week break between stopping fluoxetine and starting an MAOI, and several weeks before starting any other antidepressant.

   The other SSRIs have a shorter half-life and do not require as long a wash-out before another medication can be started.

2. *Sertraline (Zoloft)* is typically started at 50 mg/day, and a typical dose is between 50 and 200 mg/day. Its half-life is around 26 hours, but varies considerably from one person to the next. All the SSRIs can raise the serum level of other medications,

but Zoloft may do this a bit less than the others.

3. *Paroxetine (Paxil)*. A typical dose of paroxetine is 20 mg/day, with a range of 10–50 mg/day. It has been suggested that side effects of paroxetine include a lower incidence of nervousness and sleep problems than the other SSRIs. Paroxetine is also the least expensive medication in this group. All the SSRIs can raise the serum level of many other medications, but paroxetine (along with sertraline) may do this a bit less than the others.

4. *Fluvoxamine (Luvox)* is an SSRI antidepressant that has been approved for use (along with clomipramine) for the treatment of obsessive compulsive disorder. It is usually started at 50 mg before bed, with a normal dose range of 100–300 mg/day. It appears to have a somewhat different side effect profile than the other SSRIs, which makes it preferred for some patients. It usually is more sedating and less likely to cause agitation than the others. As with the other SSRIs, headaches, nausea, tiredness, and sexual problems are common side effects.

5. *Venlafaxine (Effexor)* is a bit different from the other SSRIs because it blocks the reuptake of both serotonin and norepinephrine without blocking other neurotransmitters. There is little research comparing its effectiveness to the other SSRIs, but it has been suggested that venlafaxine may be effective in some patients who have not been helped by the pure serotonergic antidepressants because it affects two different chemical systems involved in depression.

   Venlafaxine may cause high blood pressure more often than the other SSRIs, especially at doses above 225 mg/day, but it causes less interference with the metabolism of other drugs. Fluoxetine can interfere with the metabolism of venlafaxine, however, and if a client is switching from one to the other, he or she should start with a very low dose and increase very gradually over a number of weeks.

Side Effects

SSRIs have different side effect profiles than the older tricyclic antidepressants. SSRIs tend to cause weight loss rather than weight gain and they tend to be activating rather than sedating, although both weight gain and sedation occur in some clients. As a group, they also are very well tolerated with relatively few side effects, although some clients complain of increased anxiety, nausea, and headaches. Sexual dysfunction, both difficulty having an orgasm and decreased libido, is a fairly common dose-related side effect of this class of medication. Suicide is always a risk for depressed clients who are beginning to come out of their depression and become activated, but there is no evidence that Prozac or other medications in this class increase this risk. They are much less lethal after an overdose than tricyclic antidepressants and have fewer cardiac side effects.

Drug-drug interactions

New-generation antidepressants interact with a number of other medications in complicated and often dangerous ways.

1. *P450 enzyme inhibition.* SSRIs can interfere with the metabolism of many common medications. Many different medications are broken apart and made harmless in the liver by a set of enzymes called the P450 system. All SSRIs interfere with these enzymes to varying degrees, which in turn can cause normally prescribed doses of other medications to build up to dangerous levels. To further complicate matters, different SSRIs interfere with different enzymes in the P450 system, which means that different SSRIs interact with different medications. Paroxetine and fluoxetine cause the most inhibition of the enzyme that metabolizes tricyclic antidepressants, and they have the largest potential for causing dangerous increases in serum levels when they are given along with medications like desipramine. Fluvoxamine interferes most with the enzyme that metabolizes clozapine. Sertraline, fluoxetine, and nefazodone interfere with the enzyme that metabolizes the common antihistamines terfenadine (Seldane) and astemizole (Hismanal), which can lead to dangerous increases in these normally safe medications.

   There are more than 30 specific enzymes in the P450 system, and no one can keep all of the interactions in mind. What is important to remember is that different SSRIs interfere with different parts of this system, and that the serum level of many common medications can increase dramatically when the common medication is given along with an SSRI. Most pharmacists have computer programs that can look for interactions among a list of medications that a patient is taking.

2. *Serotonin syndrome.* This is most common and most dangerous when an SSRI is prescribed with an MAOI antidepressant, although it can occur as an interaction with other drugs or even as a side effect of an SSRI alone. Symptoms include confusion, agitation, sweating, increased reflexes, myoclonus (sudden jerking movements), shivering, tremor, problems with coordination, fever, and diarrhea. Serotonin syndrome can also occur when SSRIs are taken along with a number of other medications, including dextromethorphan, a very common ingredient in cough medications.

Drug Withdrawal

People who abruptly stop the SSRIs (and most of the other antidepressants) may have uncomfortable but not dangerous withdrawal symptoms for up to several days or even longer. These withdrawal symptoms can include dizziness, headaches, nausea, vivid dreams, sleep problems, irritability, and paresthesias (sense of prickling or burning of the skin). These withdrawal symptoms are more common with shorter-activating medication, such as paroxetine and fluvoxamine, and much less common with sertraline and fluoxetine.

Miscellaneous "New-Generation" Antidepressants

1. *Bupropion (Wellbutrin)* is reputed to have fewer side effects than the older antidepressants. It has fewer anticholinergic side effects (dry mouth, blurred vision, constipation) than the tricyclic antidepressants. It causes fewer blood pressure problems, and has less effect on the electrical activity of the heart. It is also an activating rather than a sedating medication, and

does not seem to cause the weight gain associated with tricyclics. Further, it has fewer sexual side effects and is safer than tricyclics if taken in overdose. Other than dangerous interactions with MAOIs, it has relatively few drug-drug side effects.

Bupropion's introduction was delayed because of a high incidence of seizures in several clients, all of whom had anorexia. Bupropion's side effects include a higher incidence of seizures, estimated at four times that of most other antidepressants. The seizure incidence is dose-related and increases tenfold when the dose is increased to 450–600 mg/day.

A normal dose of bupropion is around 300 mg/day, usually divided into three 100 mg doses. To decrease the risk of seizure, no single dose should exceed 150 mg. Bupropion is typically started at 100 mg twice a day, and increased no sooner than every 3 days.

A longer-acting version of bupropion (Wellbutrin SR) is now available. Up to 400 mg of the long-acting bupropion can be given as 200 mg twice a day, rather than taking the medication three times a day, as regular bupropion at that dose requires. The incidence of seizures is reported to be lower with the long-acting bupropion. The longer-acting bupropion has lower peak levels of medication and therefore affects the dopamine system somewhat less than the standard bupropion. Some clients may not respond as well with the long-acting medication, but the increased safety, increased convenience, and decreased risk make the long-acting form the choice of most clients.

Bupropion has also been effective in helping people stop smoking. It seems to stop the craving associated with smoking withdrawal and works best when given along with a nicotine patch and as part of a smoking cessation program. One typically sets a "stop smoking day" 7–10 days after starting bupropion. Patients participating in smoking cessation studies started at 150 mg/day for 3 days and then increased to 150 twice a day.

2. *Trazodone (Desyrel)* is probably less effective than other anti-

depressants as a primary treatment for depression but still has a useful role. Trazodone is very sedating and is often given at night as a mild, safe, non-addicting sleep aid. In fact, trazodone is sometimes prescribed to help clients overcome sleep difficulties caused by activating antidepressants like Prozac. Trazodone is a short-acting medication with a half-life of about 3½ hrs. This means that for most people there is little sedation, or hang-over, the next day if it is taken at night.

The most serious problem with trazodone is priapism (very painful, long-lasting erections of the penis), which has required surgery and led to permanent impotence in a few clients. Any man prescribed trazodone should be warned to stop taking the medication if he experiences any unusual or prolonged erections.

Trazodone has almost no anticholinergic effect, although it does cause dry mouth through a different mechanism. Trazodone is also less likely than the tricyclic antidepressants to potentiate heart block (block of electrical impulses between different parts of the heart) in clients with preexisting heart disease, although it can increase heart irritability and increase abnormal heartbeats in some people with preexisting heart disease. Trazodone is much safer in overdoses than the older medications and causes less orthostatic hypotension.

A typical dose of trazodone is 150–600 mg/day.

3. *Nefazodone (Serzone)* is similar to trazodone but appears to be more effective because it has several active metabolites that are more effective antidepressants than the parent medication. It works through a somewhat different mechanism than any of the other antidepressants.

   Nefazodone has relatively few side effects in most people. Some people report sedation, nausea, dizziness, and anticholinergic side effects including dry mouth, constipation, and blurred vision. As with the SSRIs, patients can experience headaches and nausea. Nervousness, weight loss, and palpitations all seem less common with nefazodone, and the incidence of sexual side effects also appears lower. It has some significant drug-drug interactions, specifically with the antihistamines terfenadine (Seldane) and astemizole (Hismanal) and with cisapride (Propulsid), which is a common medication for gastrointestinal disorders, such as severe chronic nausea, heartburn, or gastric reflux.

Nefazodone seems most effective in a 300–600 mg/day dose range. Because some of the metabolites have a short half-life, twice-a-day dosing is indicated. It is generally started at 50–100 mg twice a day and then increased.

4. *Mirtazapine (Remeron)* is a new antidepressant that seems to work by stimulating the release of both serotonin and norepinephrine. Its effect on these two systems seems to change according to the dose. It is often more sedating in lower doses than in higher doses, which means that clients may have fewer side effects if it is started at full dose rather than gradually increased the way most medications are. Mirtazapine seems to help the anxiety and the sleep problems common to depression and has minimal sexual side effects.

   Side effects include sedation, increased appetite, weight gain, and dizziness. It has relatively mild anticholinergic side effects, including dry mouth and constipation. It seems to have relatively few drug-drug interactions and seems relatively safe in overdose. According to early research, slightly more than one person in a thousand stops or decreases production of white blood cells.

   Mirtazapine is typically started at 15 mg before bed and can be increased to 45 mg.

Tricyclic Antidepressants

Most of the antidepressants used prior to the last few years were "tricyclics" (having a three-ring molecular structure). They include amitriptyline (Elavil), nortriptyline (Pamelor), desipramine (Norpramin), and doxepin (Sinequan).

Specifics of Use

For anyone under 16 or over 40 or anyone who has a history

of heart problems, a preliminary EKG is required before starting a tricyclic antidepressant. If there is any possibility of heart disease, a medical clearance should be obtained as well. The usual starting dose for imipramine (Tofranil) and amitriptyline (Elavil) is 50–75 mg/day for 2–3 days. If there are no serious side effects, gradually increase the dose to 150–300 mg/day. It takes from 5 days to 3 weeks for these medications to be effective, and a reasonable clinical trial is at least 3 weeks of medication in doses above 150 mg/day. After the dose is stabilized, most or all of the medication can be given right before bedtime to minimize the sedative and other side effects and to insure a good night's sleep.

It is now possible to determine how much medication is actually present in the body. One client may have 10 times the serum level of another client taking the same daily dose of medication. For some medications, such as nortriptyline, there appears to be a "therapeutic window"; that is, serum levels within a certain range (50–150 mg/ml) are more effective than levels below or above this range. For other antidepressants, lower levels seem ineffective while higher levels are, except for their higher side effects, okay. While we now can measure the serum levels of most anitdepressants, there still is too little research for us to fully understand what the serum levels mean and how much medication is too much.

The serotonergic antidepressants like Prozac can interfere with the metabolism of many other medications, including tricyclic antidepressants. This means that if a medication like Prozac is prescribed along with a tricyclic such as desipramine, a normal dose of desipramine can rapidly increase to a dangerous serum level. The same thing can happen if a patient is rapidly switched from Prozac to desipramine.

Side Effects

1. *Tricyclic antidepressants are all extremely dangerous when taken as an overdose,* and a severely depressed, potentially suicidal client should not be given more than a week's supply

of a tricyclic antidepressants without careful consideration. All of the newer antidepressants, such as venlafaxine (Effexor), fluoxetine (Prozac), and sertraline (Zoloft), are much safer if taken as an overdose.

2. *The tricyclic antidepressants potentiate the effect of alcohol,* and a few drinks may make a client on these medications more intoxicated than he or she would normally get. In addition, alcohol increases the lethality of antidepressants, and a normally nonlethal overdose may become lethal if combined with alcohol.

3. *Anticholinergic side effects are common.* All the traditional, tricyclic antidepressants block the action of acetylcholine and produce the kind of autonomic side effects (side effects related to the involuntary part of the nervous system responsible for basic system regulation) typical of other anticholinergic medications. These include dry mouth, blurred vision, constipation, and, in rare cases, urinary retention, heart palpitations, or tachycardia (speeding pulse) and increased sweating. These medications can, on rare occasions, aggravate certain kinds of glaucoma (increased pressure in the eyeball) and eye pain, which can be helped by special eye drops.

   Anticholinergic medications can also cause confusion and delirium, especially in elderly people who may be taking a number of different medications with anticholinergic side effects.

4. *Cardiovascular side effects include orthostatic hypotension (drop in blood pressure when the person stands up), increased pulse, and EKG changes.* The most serious of these side effects are sudden cardiac arrhythmias (irregularities of the heart beat) or heart block, when the electrical impulses cannot spread through the heart normally. Sudden death has been reported, but it is extremely rare. Overall, the effects on the heart are very complicated and not all bad. The tricyclic antidepressants (e.g., amitriptyline, desipramine) act on the heart very much like quinidine, a medication used to stabilize cer-

tain kinds of heartbeat irregularities. In fact, a client with heart problems who normally requires quinidine can often reduce or eliminate his or her dose if he or she begins taking one of these antidepressants.

5. *Neurological complications are fairly rare.* Grand mal seizures can be caused by all the tricyclic antidepressants. Two newer antidepressants, bupropion (Wellbutrin) and maprotiline (Ludiomil), seem to have a somewhat higher incidence of seizures than the tricyclics, while all the other newer antidepressants have a much lower seizure frequency. Other side effects of the tricyclics include drowsiness, slurred speech, and hand tremor. Like any other medication with anticholinergic properties, these medications can also cause confusion or even delirium that may be difficult to distinguish from a psychotic episode.

6. *Weight gain is a common problem caused by all of the tricyclic and MAOI antidepressants.* The newer antidepressants, including bupropion (Wellbutrin) and the serotonin-blocking antidepressants (fluoxetine and sertraline), do not normally cause weight gain and may cause some weight loss.

7. *Many antidepressants, including the tricyclics, can cause decreased libido and impotence.* They can also block menstrual periods, although this seems less common. Decreasing the dose or switching antidepressants may solve these problems.

8. *All antidepressant medications can trigger a manic episode* in some susceptible people. This may be more likely with the tricyclics than with the newer antidepressants. In addition, some schizophrenic clients are reported to become more disorganized or more paranoid when taking antidepressants. These medications can also cause some clients to start "rapid cycling," to have rapid mood swings more than once a month.

9. *Various allergies can also occur,* and any client on any medication who reports a new rash should have it investigated. Also, as with the antipsychotic medications, agranulocytosis

(sudden block in white blood cell production) has been reported. If a client has a sore throat, sudden chills, or fever, a physician should be alerted and a complete blood count (CBC) should be drawn immediately.

10. *Abrupt withdrawal of these medications sometimes produces nausea, vomiting, abdominal cramps, diarrhea, chills, insomnia, and anxiety lasting 3–5 days.* This withdrawal is not medically dangerous but can be uncomfortable. These medications usually should be withdrawn gradually over several weeks or even longer, especially if the person has been taking the medication for some time.

11. *While these medications usually help sleep, occasionally they produce nightmares.* This can be controlled by lowering the dose, taking the medication earlier in the day, or taking it in divided doses. Agitation and nervousness are uncommon but have been reported.

Monoamine Oxidase Inhibitors (MAOIs)

MAOIs include phenelzine (Nardil) and tranylcypromine (Parnate). They block the action of the enzyme that deactivates neurotransmitters with a single amine group, hence their name mono (one) amine oxidase inhibitors. They have always been widely used in England, and have been used more frequently in the United States over the past few years. Some clients who have not responded to other medications will respond to MAOIs. MAOIs seem to be particularly useful in clients with "atypical depression." These clients often have problems with anxiety and agoraphobic symptoms, may have weight gain instead of the more common weight loss, and may sleep too much instead of too little. Some researchers suggest that clients with "hysteroid dysphoria," a vague constellation of symptoms and marked sensitivity to rejection, may respond specifically to MAOIs. Others feel that clients with bulimia and agoraphobia may respond better to these medications than to traditional antidepressants.

Specifics of Use

Clients must be off all other antidepressants for at least 10 days before starting a MAOI (clients must be off fluoxetine [Prozac] for 5 weeks). Similarly, if a client switches from one MAOI to another there must be at least a 10-day medication-free period. The dose of the medication is gradually increased over a week or two, and as with the other antidepressants it usually takes 3 weeks or longer for the medication to be effective.

Side Effects

1. *The most common serious side effect is a hypertensive crisis* (very rapid, very high, and dangerous elevation of blood pressure). This reaction is caused by an interaction between the MAOI and foods containing tyramine, or between the MAOI and medications that have sympathomimetic effects (effects on the sympathetic nervous system). The MAOIs work by interfering with the enzyme that breaks apart certain neurotransmitters. This same enzyme also breaks apart tyramine, an amino acid that naturally occurs in certain foods. Since the MAOI keeps this tyramine from being deactivated, it can rapidly accumulate to high levels and cause the increase in blood pressure.

   The symptoms of a hypertensive crisis include a severe headache, heart palpitations, nausea and vomiting, unexplained nose bleed, and chest pain. A blood pressure check can quickly determine whether or not there is a problem. Such crises are rare, especially if clients are compliant with the food restrictions, but they can lead to strokes and other catastrophes.

   Foods that have high levels of tyramine and must be avoided include:

   - Aged cheeses (essentially everything except bland American cheese)
   - Smoked or pickled fish
   - Chicken liver

- Broad beans (fava beans)
- Chianti and other red wines
- Tap and German beers
- Sauerkraut
- Sausage, salami, and other aged meat
- Dried, salted fish
- Any food that is not fresh

In addition, a large number of additional foods, including chocolate, yogurt, and sour cream, have moderate levels of tyramine and can cause a reaction in some people, especially if eaten in large amounts. A variety of aged foods, such as overripe bananas, can cause problems, as can monosodium glutamate, soy sauce, and meat tenderizer.

2. *MAOIs interact with a large number of other medications,* often in dangerous ways. For example, extremely dangerous interactions occur when Demerol is taken by someone also taking an MAOI. Dextromethorphan, found in many over-the-counter cough medications, is also dangerous. A potentially fatal "serotonin reaction" can occur when MAOIs are given along with SSRIs and other antidepressants that affect serotonin. Because Prozac has a long half-life, a person should not take an MAOI until he or she has been off Prozac for at least 5 weeks.

   Many non-prescription cold and allergy medications and asthma medications can cause a hypertensive reaction, as can stimulants such as amphetamines and cocaine.

   Clients taking MAOIs are strongly advised to check with their doctor or pharmacist about medication interactions before taking any other medication, whether prescribed or over-the-counter.

   Clients taking MAOIs should let all treating physicians, dentists, and other health care providers know exactly what medications they are taking. Some form of emergency notification, such as a card in their wallet or I.D. bracelet, is also a useful precaution.

3. *MAOIs can also cause orthostatic hypotension* (drop in blood

pressure when the client stands up quickly). This can cause temporary dizziness or even fainting, and often the use of the medication must be limited.

4. *MAOIs are activating rather than sedating medications for most people.* This is often an advantage, since they usually do not cause the sedation that is common with other antidepressants, but this activating effect can interfere with sleep. Most people prefer to take these medications early in the day rather than at night, when tricyclics are usually taken. At times it is useful to give low-dose trazodone at night if sleep disturbance

TABLE 9. *Profiles of Antidepressants*

Antidepressant	Anticholinergic effect	Sedative effect	Inhibition of Reuptake	
			Norepinephrine	Serotonin
TRICYCLIC/TERTIARY AMINES				
amitriptyline (Elavil)	+ + + +	+ + + +	+ +	+ + + +
clomipramine (Anafranil)	+ + +	+ + +	+ +	+ + + +
doxepin (Adapin, Sinequan)	+ +	+ + +	+	+ +
imipramine (Tofranil)	+ +	+ +	+ + + +	+
trimipramine (Surmontil)	+ +	+ + +	+	+
TRICYCLIC SECONDARY AMINES				
amoxapine (Asendin)	+ + +	+ +	+ + +	+ +
desipramine (Norpramin, Pertofrane)	+	+	+ + + +	+ +
nortriptyline (Aventyl, Pamelor)	+ +	+ +	+ +	+ + +
protriptyline (Vivactil)	+ + +	+	+ + + +	+ +
NEW ANTIDEPRESSANTS				
bupropion (Wellbutrin)	+ +	+ +	0/+	0/+
fluoxetine (Prozac)	0/+	0/+	0/+	+ + + +
fluvoxamine (Luvox)	0	0/+	0/+	+ + + +
maprotiline (Ludiomil)	+ +	+ +	+ + +	+/0
nefazodone (Serzone)	0/+	+ +	0/+	+ + + +
paroxetine (Paxil)	0/+	+	0/+	+ + + +
sertraline (Zoloft)	0	0/+	0/+	+ + + +
trazodone (Desyrel)	+	+ + +	0	+ + +
venlafaxine (Effexor)	0	0/+	+ + +	+ + +

KEY: + Slight + + Moderate + + + High + + + + Highest 0 None
Adapted from *Drug Facts and Comparisons*, 1997, St. Louis, MO: Facts and Comparisons.

is a significant problem. Some people do get sedated from the MAOIs, and feeling lethargic a few hours after taking the medication is not uncommon.

5. *Other side effects are usually less of a problem and less common.* Constipation or diarrhea is sometimes reported, as is dry mouth, transient impotence, skin rash, and blurred vision, despite the fact that MAOIs are not anticholinergic. Serious liver toxicity is rare, but has been reported with phenelzine (Nardil).

6. *As with other antidepressants, problems can occur if an MAOI is stopped abruptly.* Withdrawal symptoms include confusion, irritability, agitation, depression, and manic symptoms.

Deciding Which Antidepressant to Use

All of the antidepressants currently available seem equally effective, although a particular medication may be dramatically more effective than another for a particular individual. Unfortunately, there is no way to be certain about which medication will work for which client. Physicians are often inclined to select certain antidepressants because they are familiar with them. It is reasonable to select the medication with a side effect profile least troublesome to the particular client. The main side effects to consider in choosing a medication are degree of sedation, degree of anticholinergic activity, cardiovascular side effects (including orthostatic hypotension), and sexual side effects. For example, desipramine is only mildly sedating and has relatively few anticholinergic side effects (dry mouth, blurred vision, etc.). This might be a good medication to choose for clients who have had problems with sedation or blurred vision. Fluoxetine (Prozac) might be the medication of choice if no sedation can be tolerated. Fluoxetine usually does not cause weight gain, but increases anxiety in some susceptible clients. Doxepin (Sinequan), on the other hand, is very sedating, and for clients with insomnia this medication's sedative "side effect" might be useful if there is little risk of overdose. If sexual side effects are

TABLE 10. *Reported Incidence of Side Effects of New Antidepressants (percentage reported over placebo)*

Side Effect	Fluoxetine	Sertraline	Paroxetine	Venlafaxine	Nefazodone	Buproprion
Headache	4.8	1.3	0.3	1	3	3.5
Nervousness	10.3	4.4	4.9	12	-	13.9
Tremors	5.5	8	6.4	4	1	13.5
Insomnia	6.7	7.6	7.1	8	2	5.3
Drowsiness	5.9	7.5	14.3	14	11	0.3
Dizziness	4	5	7.8	12	23	6.8
Nausea	11	14.3	16.4	26	11	4.0
Diarrhea	5.3	8.4	4	1	1	-
Dry mouth	3.5	7	6	11	12	9.2
Sweating	4.6	5.5	8.8	9	-	7.7
Decreased orgasm	?	13.3	12.9	12	?	-
Decreased libido	1.9	1.5	3.3	2	1.7	-

Adapted from "Comparison of the Tolerability of Buproprion, Fluoxetine, Imipramine, Nefazodone, Paroxetine, Sertraline, and Venlafaxine," by S. Preskorn, 1995, *Journal of Clinical Psychiatry*, 56, p. 18.

of concern, bupropion (Wellbutrin) or nefazodone (Serzone) might be the best choice.

When the first antidepressant does not work and a second medication is being considered, it makes sense to choose a second medication as different as possible from the first, although there are few hard data to support this theory. All six types of antidepressants (tricyclics, MAOIs, SSRIs, bupropion, nefazodone, mirtazapine) have somewhat different mechanisms of action. Occasionally, a client will respond to one medication and not another even though the medications are of the same type.

Mood-stabilizing medications, such as lithium, are often used to increase the effectiveness of an antidepressant if the antidepressant alone is not fully effective. A number of other augmentation strategies also work well, including combining different antidepressants with different mechanisms of action, using thyroid hormone even when there appears to be normal thyroid function, and adding pindolol (a beta-blocker) to an antidepressant. While there appears to be anecdotal support for these strategies, there is little controlled research demonstrating which of these strategies is most effective for whom.

6

Mood-Stabilizing Medications

The classic mood stabilizer is lithium. First used in 1949 as an anti-manic treatment, it was the first modern "wonder drug" in psychiatry. In addition to lithium, a number of medications traditionally used to control seizures are now used as mood stabilizers. Valproate and valproic acid (Depakote) and carbamazepine (Tegretol) are now widely used. Several new anticonvulsants also seem to have mood-stabilizing properties and are used solely for those properties. Medications called calcium channel blockers that are typically used to control angina might also have a role to play in the treatment of mood disorders, but data on this are less clear.

Mood stabilizers are not "uppers" or "downers" or simple antidepressants. They stabilize both the highs and the lows of some clients' mood swings. Mood swings do not always disappear, but they often become less frequent and less severe. In general, mood stabilizers treat classic bipolar disorder, with mood swings occurring less than twice a year, better than they treat rapid cycling disorder or other more atypical mood disorders.

Lithium

Indications for Use

Lithium is the medication of choice for the prophylactic control of the manic-depressive client. It decreases the frequency and severity of the manic episodes, but it does not necessarily eliminate them in all clients. It is also useful in aborting the acute manic attack and is often used in combination with one of the antipsychotic medications. The antipsychotic slows the client down to a manageable level while the lithium aborts the manic attack itself.

There is also increasing evidence that lithium is useful in schizoaffective disorder and even in some agitated or aggressive schizophrenic clients. Clients who are hyperactive and have pressured speech should be considered as potential lithium candidates, even if they carry a schizophrenic diagnosis. A certain percentage of lithium responders previously have been given a diagnosis of schizophrenia. These clients may have carried a schizophrenic diagnosis for many years, and they may have all the first-rank symptoms of schizophrenia. It makes sense to seriously consider a trial of lithium for schizophrenic clients not responding well to more traditional therapy and those who are irritable, angry, or aggressive, all of which are affective symptoms. Whenever a medication is first begun and especially when initiating such trials, it is important to remember that they are just that—trials. The medication should be started and continued for a specified period of time, usually 4–6 weeks, and target symptoms that were clearly identified before the trial should be followed.

A family history of manic-depressive disorder, depression, or suicide increases the probability that the client is a lithium responder, and it is suggested that a family history of alcoholism might also be a positive sign. A client who reports experiencing depressions and "highs," bouts of excessively spending, or frequent, impulsive marriages should be considered as possibly having mania.

Lithium is also helpful in preventing the depressive side of manic-depressive disease and recurrent depression. Recent research has indicated that combining lithium and antidepressants is very effective in treating some clients who have never responded to antidepressants alone. Many clients with borderline and other personality disorders show marked and at times rapid mood changes, from sad to elated and back again. For some clients, lithium or one of the other mood stabilizers will help decrease the number of these mood fluctuations.

Lithium also has been effective in some clients with explosive, uncontrollable anger that does not leave time for the client to consider the consequences of his behavior.

Specifics of Use

Before starting lithium, a serum BUN (blood urea nitrogen) and serum creatinine should be obtained to determine that the client's kidneys are working properly. Lithium is excreted by the kidneys, and if they are not working properly the lithium can rapidly build up to toxic levels. An EKG is suggested by some experts but is probably unnecessary, unless there is concern about heart disease. Some experts suggest a creatinine clearance test as well, but this requires collecting all of a person's urine over 24 hours, which is quite cumbersome, expensive, and usually impossible in the community. Following serum creatinine over the course of lithium therapy is a reasonably safe way to detect early kidney damage. A yearly urinalysis may give some information about the kidneys' ability to concentrate urine, but is not part of most protocols. Though there was early concern about lithium and kidney damage, such damage seems extremely rare. A lab test for thyroid function taken before starting lithium and regularly thereafter is also often recommended.

Start by giving 600–1200 mg/day of lithium carbonate in divided doses. Lithium carbonate usually comes in 300 mg capsules, so a typical dose is three to four capsules a day. Lithium was once given two or three times a day because of concern of toxicity and side effects. Recently, it has become apparent that most clients do well taking the entire dose at one time, usually at mealtime to decrease gastrointestinal side effects.

Follow with serum lithium levels and adjust the dose so that the lithium level in the blood is 0.6–1.2 meq/l. The textbooks used to suggest that lithium levels be 0.8–1.2 meq/l. Recent research has suggested that clients have fewer relapses if their lithium is kept between .8 and 1.0 meq/l than if their level is allowed to drop to the 0.4–0.6 meq/l range. Unfortunately, they also have poorer compliance and more side effects at the higher levels. While there is some increased risk of relapse at the lower dose, for some clients the decrease in side effects may make this risk worthwhile. Most clients require 600–1,800 mg/day to maintain their serum lithium level within this therapeutic range. Older clients and clients with brain damage generally require less lithium and, in fact, may become toxic on normal doses. Usually, as clients end a manic episode, less medication is needed to maintain the same serum medication level. Clients who have had a stable lithium level while manic may become toxic if they continue to take the same amount of lithium after they calm down. Conversely, clients going into a manic episode will frequently need to increase their daily lithium dose to maintain a therapeutic serum lithium level.

After a client seems stable on a given dose of lithium, blood levels should be measured at least every six months. Blood levels change during the day, peaking several hours after the client takes a dose and dropping slowly until the next dose. It is important, therefore, to standardize when the blood sample is drawn. A serum level of .6 meq/l 12 hours after a dose means something different from the same level 24 hours after a dose. Standard serum levels should always be taken 12 hours after a normal dose of medication is taken. A client receiving divided doses of lithium should have his or her lithium level checked before taking his or her morning dose, which should be about 12 hours after the evening dose was taken.

Some of the side effects from lithium can be treated. Mild diarrhea can be treated by over-the-counter medications, such as Kaopectate. A fine intention tremor can be treated with low-dose propranolol, which is relatively safe, easy to use, and effective. Still, using one medication to treat the side effects of another only makes sense when the tremor is causing some problem or discomfort. If increased urination becomes a serious problem for the client, because it is either dehydrating or so frequent that it is interfering with the client's life, hydrochlorothiazide may be prescribed. This is a diuretic that normally causes people to urinate more but works paradoxically on clients suffering from increased urination because of lithium. There is some concern that hydrochlorothiazide may increase the risk of kidney damage from lithium, and it is only used when the increased urinary frequency is severe. Hydrochlorothiazide increases most clients' serum lithium levels, potentially to toxic levels. To prevent lithium toxicity, the dose of lithium is usually decreased at the same time that hydrochlorothiazide is started, and serum lithium levels are monitored carefully. Hydrochlorothiazide also causes potassium loss, which needs to be monitored.

Alcoholic clients on lithium present a special problem because they may become dehydrated during drinking binges, thereby secondarily increasing their serum lithium levels enough to become toxic. The resulting acute organic brain syndrome might be from lithium as well as alcohol. This is rarely a problem because these clients seldom take their medications while drinking. However, lithium toxicity should be considered for anyone who is drunk and/or dehydrated while on lithium.

Side Effects

1. *Effects on the kidney.* Lithium is excreted by the kidneys and preexisting kidney disease (determined by BUN and serum creatinine tests) can allow a dangerous buildup of the medication in a short time. Increased fluid intake and urination are common in most clients on lithium because of its direct effect on the kidneys, causing a syndrome called nephrogenic diabetes insipides. In some rare cases, this increased urination may be severe enough to cause serious dehydration. For almost all individuals, these kidney effects are more inconvenient than dangerous and correct themselves when the medication is discontinued. There has been concern that a few clients on long-term lithium therapy may incur permanent, irreversible, and potentially life-threatening kidney damage.

No clear information about the frequency of such damage is available, except that it seems to be extremely rare and can be prevented by discontinuing lithium before the kidney damage gets too severe. All clients on lithium should have their serum creatinine measured every 6–12 months to detect early kidney damage.

2. *Thyroid effects.* Lithium is known to interfere with thyroid function and it may be useful to get a yearly TSH (thyroid-stimulating hormone) to test for this. Hypothyroidism (underactive thyroid) often develops very slowly and is easy to miss. It is very important for both clinicians and clients to be aware of early signs of thyroid dysfunction and obtain a TSH if there is any concern. Signs of decreased thyroid function include weight gain, fatigue, intolerance to cold, constipation, hoarse voice, and rough, dry skin.

3. *Common, uncomfortable side effects.* The most common side effect of lithium is a fine tremor of hands that usually begins during the first few days of treatment. Nausea, vomiting, mild abdominal pain, fatigue, and thirst are also common initially but usually disappear in a few weeks. These side effects may be decreased by giving the medication in smaller divided doses or giving it along with food so that absorption is slowed. Also common is a metallic taste, weight gain, and frequent urination. Lithium can affect the heart and causes minor changes in the EKGs of many clients. This is rarely a serious problem.

4. *Toxic side effects.* Toxic side effects of lithium, which initially look like an exaggeration of the common, nontoxic side effects, include thirst, decreased appetite, vomiting, and diarrhea. However, these can progress to confusion, coarse tremor, muscle twitching, and slurred speech. In extreme cases, the client appears drunk and has muscle twitches, nystagmus (small jerks of the eye), hyperreflexia (increased

reflexes), seizures, stupor, and eventually coma. The neurological symptoms in such cases may be present in only one side of the body or may be more severe on one side than they are on the other.

If a client taking lithium develops diarrhea or nausea, lithium intoxication should be considered and serum lithium levels obtained.

Drug-Drug Interactions

Lithium interacts with a number of commonly prescribed medications. The most common problem is a rise in the serum lithium level, at times to toxic levels, when a client initially stable on lithium begins taking an additional medication. This occurs with hydrochlorothiazide, a very common medication used for water retention and high blood pressure, and with a number of pain medications, including most of the nonsteroidal, anti-inflammatory medications like indomethacin (Indocin), phenylbutazone (Butazolidin), and possibly ibuprofen (Motrin). Aspirin and acetaminophen (Tylenol) are safe.

Use during Pregnancy

There is evidence that lithium increases the risk of serious birth defects, especially if taken during the first three months of pregnancy. This risk is high enough that women who become pregnant or who are planning to become pregnant should stop taking lithium if possible.

Laboratory Monitoring

A screen for pregnancy should be done before starting the medication, either by taking a careful history or by taking a urine test. Most textbooks suggest that a screen for kidney function be done before starting lithium. I feel that in situations where it is impossible to minimize blood draws and with a healthy person it is safe to wait to obtain an initial screen for kidney function (BUN and serum creatinine) and lithium level approximately 5 days after starting lithium. A lithium level should be obtained approximately 5–7 days after each dose change. For stable patients, a lithium level should be obtained at least every six months and a creatinine level every year. All lithium levels should be drawn approximately 12 hours after the last dose of lithium.

People taking lithium over time may have a decrease in thyroid function. The standard protocol is to test for this before starting lithium and then every year or so. However, if I am trying to minimize tests I simply watch for symptoms of thyroid problems, such as weight gain, depression, a sense of sluggishness, problems tolerating cold, dry skin, and a persistently hoarse voice. If I notice any of these symptoms, I order a TSH to assess thyroid at that time.

Valproate, Valproic Acid, and Divalproex Sodium (Depakene or Depakote)

Depakote is divalproex sodium, which is a compound of valproate and valproic acid. Depakene is just valproic acid. The terms valproate, valproic acid, and divalproex sodium are used interchangeably and all are transformed to the exact same chemical in the body, although formally they are slightly different chemicals. When someone refers to a pill of valproate or valproic acid, he or she is simply using shorthand for the term divalproex sodium.

Indications for Use

Divalproex sodium was originally developed as an anticonvulsant, but it is now in widespread use as a mood stabilizer. Both divalproex sodium and lithium carbonate are considered first medications of choice for treatment of manic-depressive illness. Lithium carbonate has been used longer, we have more information about its effectiveness, and it is much cheaper than divalproex sodium. Divalproex sodium can be started at a full dose essentially from the beginning and seems to work more rapidly. Both medications have their own side effects, but for many people the side effects of divalproex sodium are easier to live with than those of lithium.

Divalproex sodium becomes the medication of choice (over lithium) when the symptoms or illness course do not fit into a classic manic-depressive pattern. Divalproex sodium is the medication of choice for people who are rapid cycling (having four or more episodes of mania or depression a year), have extreme mood instability, who have a seizure disorder or a history of seizures, or who have any history of brain damage.

Divalproex sodium is also used to increase the effectiveness of antidepressants and to treat rage reactions (uncontrollable anger).

Specifics for Use

Valproic acid is typically started with 250 mg tablets two or three times a day and increased by 250 mg every two to three days until the normal 1,000–1,500 mg/day range is reached. It is also safe and well tolerated, however, when begun essentially at a full dose, usually figured at 15–20 mg/kg. For example, a 220 lb. person (100 kg) can be safely started on 1,500–2,000 mg/day in divided doses. Effective serum concentrations are generally considered to be between 45 and 125 µg/l. This is the serum level needed to prevent seizures; there is much less research on the serum level needed for valproic acid to be an effective mood stabilizer.

It is suggested that liver function tests be obtained every 6–12 months, and serum levels every 6 months, although given the very low frequency of liver problems in adults it is unclear if this is always necessary.

Side Effects

In general, valproate is well tolerated and allows many people a greater sense of well-being and less restriction of creativity than is sometimes reported with lithium.

1. *Common side effects* include weight gain, nausea, vomiting, and indigestion. Depakote (a compound of valproic acid and sodium valproate) is packaged in a coated, time-release pill that seems to cause less gastrointestinal upset than Depakene (valproic acid alone). Sedation has been reported, although this is less common than with carbamazepine. Tremor is listed as a side effect but also seems rare. Hair loss is rare but can be a serious problem for some people. However, hair growth usually resumes even if the medication is continued and may be helped with selenium and zinc mineral supplemention.
2. *Serious side effects* are very rare, but deaths have been reported. While valproic acid has been associated with serious liver toxicity in children, this is extremely rare in adults. Valproic acid has also been reported to interfere with the ability to make white blood cells (agranulocytosis), although this seems significantly less common than with carbamazepine.

Use during Pregnancy

Valproate is associated with birth defects, primarily neural tube defects, when taken in the first trimester of the pregnancy.

Women starting valproate should be given a pregnancy test or carefully asked about the possibility of being pregnant.

Laboratory Monitoring

A screen for pregnancy should be done before starting the medication, either by taking a careful history or by taking a urine test. I get a WBC (white blood count) with differential and liver tests at the time of the first blood level, usually 5-7 days after starting the medication. I will get another WBC and liver function test in a month or two if I need another serum level, but if I have no clinical concern I may go up to six months for the next WBC and liver function tests, with yearly monitoring after that.

Carbamazepine (Tegretol)

Indications for Use

There is good evidence that carbamazepine (Tegretol) is useful in some manic-depressive clients or clients with manic-type mood swings who do not respond well to lithium or valproic acid or who cannot tolerate the side effects of these other medications. Carbamazepine can be used along with both lithium and valproic acid. It seems particularly useful for clients with atypical illness or rapid cycling manic-depressive disorder, with more than two episodes a year. It has also been used successfully in certain clients with very resistant depressions, usually in combination with other medications.

Carbamazepine is also being used in a variety of other conditions where lithium and valproic acid have been ineffective. Some people with schizophrenia whose ongoing affective lability makes stabilization difficult respond well to either lithium or carbamazepine in combination with an antipsychotic medication. Some clients with aggressive or violent outbursts also seem to respond to carbamazepine or one of the other mood-stabilizing medications. It was once thought that some kind of occult seizure disorder caused these outbursts, but carbamazepine seems to be effective in clients who have no evidence of any kind of seizures.

Specifics of Use

Carbamazepine is usually started at 100–200 mg twice a day, and the dose is increased until the serum level is 5–12 µg/l. Some people who appear confused or sedated, despite having a normal serum level, have a buildup of an active metabolite of carbamazepine called 10,11 epoxide. This, too, can be measured if there is any clinical concern. It takes approximately 5 days for a dose change to fully show up in a serum level. Carbamazepine induces liver enzymes. That is, the liver gets used to breaking it down, which makes the level tend to drop over the first six weeks or so, even if the same dose is taken. (Alcohol does the same thing, which is one of the reasons seasoned drinkers can drink more without getting as drunk.)

Side Effects of Carbamazepine

Generally carbamazepine is well tolerated and produces less weight gain, hair loss, and tremor than valproic acid, and less memory impairment and tremor than lithium. The drawbacks of carbamazepine include increased sedation, a slightly higher incidence of serious side effects, and the potential to be fatal in overdose.

1 *Sedation is common,* as are a drunk-like sense of clumsiness and nausea. These side effects are dose-related and tend to get better within a few days if the person keeps taking the medication.

2. *Carbamazepine can interfere with the production of white blood cells.* Carbamazepine can cause a slight decrease in the white cell count (leukopenia). This usually develops over time, and the white count rarely drops to a dangerous level. On very rare occasions (4 cases per million patients) the body entirely stops making white blood cells (aplastic anemia). This is reversible if diagnosed in time but fatal if allowed to continue.

Any client taking carbamazepine who gets an infection, fever, sore throat, or mouth sores should immediately get a CBC (complete blood count).

Regular white blood counts are not very useful in preventing the abrupt development of agranulocytosis, but they will indicate any gradual decrease in white cell counts.

3. *Rashes are relatively common* and can on rare occasions lead to serious problems. Generally the medication does not need to be stopped if a mild rash develops, as long as there is no associated fever, bleeding, or peeling time blisters (exfoliative rash).

4. *Temporary increases in liver enzymes are fairly common.*

Generally liver function tests should be monitored, but the medication does not need to be stopped unless they are twice the normal values.

Drug-drug Interactions

Carbamazepine can interfere with the effectiveness of many oral contraceptives.

Erythromycin, cimetidine, and SSRI antidepressants can all increase the serum level of carbamazepine. Serum levels of many antipsychotics such as haloperidol are decreased when carbamazepine is started. And the combination of carbamazepine and clozapine may increase the risk of agranulocytosis.

Use during Pregnancy

Carbamazepine is associated with birth defects, especially during the first trimester.

These are similar to the birth defects caused by another anticonvulsant, phenytoin (Dilantin). Birth defects caused by carbamazepine include neural tube defects, defects in the face and skull, underdevelopment of fingernails, and developmental delay. Women starting carbamazepine should be given a pregnancy test or carefully asked about the possibility of being pregnant.

Laboratory Monitoring

A screen for pregnancy should be done before starting the medication, either by taking a careful history or by taking a urine test. The biggest danger is that carbamazepine can interfere with white blood cell production and can cause liver problems. It is important to instruct patients about the warning signs of a decrease in white blood cell production. Any patient on carbamazepine, especially during the first six months, who has a fever, sore throat, or symptoms of a flu should immediately have a white blood count obtained. Patients should also be alert to any symptoms of hepatitis, including abdominal tenderness under the right ribs.

Most texts suggest assessing white blood cell production before starting any medication. Certainly, a baseline pre-medication WBC (white blood count) can be useful. If I am trying to minimize blood tests and the client is healthy, I feel it is reasonably safe to get both the first WBC with differential and initial screen for liver problems (SGOT, SGPT, LDH) at the time the first blood level is taken, approximately 5 days after starting the medication. I get a repeat WBC every time I get a blood level, which usually is several times in the first month of treatment. I then try to get a repeat WBC with differential and liver function test at 3 months, at 6 months, and at least every 12 months thereafter. Carbamazepine auto-induces enzymes, which means that the serum level tends to drop during the first couple months and needs to be monitored more frequently at the beginning. All carbamazepine levels should be drawn approximately 12 hours after the last dose of carbamazepine.

New Mood Stabilizers in Development

Lamotrigine (Lamictal)

This new anticonvulsant that seems to be effective for people with rapid-cycling bipolar disorder, hard-to-treat mixed states, and rapid cycling caused by antidepressants. There is no research to support such use of the drug, but there are a number of anecdotal reports and controlled studies are now underway.

Specifics of Use. Generally start with 25 mg/day (12.5 mg for people on valproic acid) and increase by 25 mg every 5–7 days. Increasing the dose more rapidly seems to increase the risk of developing a rash. A typical dose is 100-200 mg/day for people on lamotrigine alone. Because of enzyme induction, a higher dose may be required if lamotrigine is taken along with carbamazepine. Because of enzyme inhibition, a lower dose is usually needed if taken with valproic acid.

Side Effects. Lamotrigine generally is well tolerated. The most problematic side effect is a rash that can progress to a potentially life-threatening condition in approximately one person in a thousand.

Anyone taking lamotrigine should be instructed to discontinue the medication immediately if a rash develops.

This seems less likely to develop if the medication is started low and increased gradually. Other possible side effects include clumsiness, dizziness, drowsiness, headaches, and nausea.

Gabapentin (Neurotin)

This new-generation anticonvulsant seems to have mood-stabilizing properties as well. As with lamotrigine, there are anecdotal case reports and research is underway but not yet published. It seems generally well tolerated and safe (even in overdose). It is also being used to treat headaches.

Specifics of Use. Gabapentin is started at 300 mg/day with a rapid titration to 900 mg/day. A typical dose range is 900–1800 mg/day, but up to 3600 mg seems safe.

Side Effects. These include tiredness, dizziness, headache, nausea, blurred or double vision, clumsiness, and tremor.

Verapamil (Calan, Isoptin)

Verapamil is in the class of medications called calcium channel blockers. These are commonly used for angina, but it has been suggested that they are useful in mania as well. The research literature on the use of these medications for mania is mixed, with some support and some negative findings.

Specifics of Use. Start with 80 mg twice a day, increasing to a maximum dose of 480 mg/day. A slow-release 240 mg tablet is also available.

Side Effects. Verapamil is generally very well tolerated and very safe. Side effects include dizziness, headache, and nausea. Irregularities of heartbeat and liver problems are rare but have been reported. Verapamil can cause a drop in blood pressure, especially in older people. There are some reports of neurotoxicity when verapamil is used in combination with lithium or carbamazepine.

7

Antianxiety and Sleeping Medications

Almost all of the central nervous system depressants, including alcohol and barbituates, have antianxiety properties and can be used as tranquilizers. Similarly, these medications all have sedative properties and can be used to aid sleep. Antianxiety medications are sometimes referred to as "minor tranquilizers" to distinguish them from the antipsychotic medications, which are sometimes called "major tranquilizers." These names are very misleading. "Minor tranquilizers" are extremely effective and not at all "minor." "Major tranquilizers" are sedating, and therefore have some tranquilizing properties, but are more accurately labeled antipsychotic medication. Antianxiety medications are also referred to as anxiolytic. Sleeping pills are referred to as hypnotics.

The most useful tranquilizers are those that have the largest antianxiety effects with the least sedation. The benzodiazepines have largely supplanted older medications like barbiturates. Benzodiazepines include diazepam (Valium), chlordiazepoxide (Librium), clonazepam (Klonopin), alprazolam (Xanax), flurazepam (Dalmane), and many others, and are much safer and less addicting than the older medications. The new medication buspirone (BuSpar) appears to be even safer and less addicting than the benzodiazepines. Eventually it may replace them in some cases, although there is strong suggestion that it is less effective. Sedating antihistamines such as diphenhydramine (Benadryl) can also be used as either an antianxiety medication or as a sleeping pill, although it is less effective and has more side effects than the benzodiazepines.

The benzodiazepines, barbiturates, and many of the other medications used as sleeping pills or antianxiety medications can be addicting and are subject to abuse. These addicting medications are all at least partially cross-tolerant (an addicted individual can replace one medication with another in that class), and withdrawal from these medications is much more medically dangerous than heroin withdrawal. Abruptly stopping the use of medications in someone who is addicted to alcohol, barbiturates, or diazepam (Valium) can result in a life-threatening convulsions. If addiction to any of these medications is a possibility in a client, medication for a gradual detoxification should be prescribed, and hospital admission may be necessary to control drug use. The sedating antihistamines, e.g., diphenhydramine (Benadryl), are subject to abuse, but are not physiologically addicting and are not cross-tolerant with the others. Buspirone (BuSpar) seems to be neither subject to abuse nor addicting.

Benzodiazepines

Benzodiazepines include diazepam (Valium), chlordiazepoxide (Librium), alprazolam (Xanax), flurazepam (Dalmane), and others. Medications in the benzodiazepine class are usually the choice when a minor tranquilizer is indicated.

Indications for Use

The benzodiazepines are most commonly used as antianxiety medications. They are relatively safe medications that are rarely lethal in an overdose, except when combined with alcohol. They have anticonvulsant properties—clonazepam (Klonopin) is regularly used as an anticonvulsant, and diazepam (Valium) can be used intravenously to stop a seizure. In those very rare instances when a client must be sedated before you know what is going on, a benzodiazepine, such as diazepam or lorazepam, is a good medication to use, as it is usually safer than antipsychotic medications like Thorazine and Haldol. Some of the benzodiazepines, e.g., alprazolam (Xanax) and clonazepam (Klonopin), have antipanic and mood-stabilizing properties.

As with all medications, the benzodiazepines should not be used without a reason and should not be continued without a reason for continuation.

Specifics of Use

1. *As an antianxiety medication*, diazepam (Valium) is commonly prescribed in 5- or 10-mg tablets up to 40 mg/day. Chlordiazepoxide (Librium) is usually prescribed in doses of 10–25 mg up to 100 mg/day. When alprazolam (Xanax) is used as an antianxiety medication, a typical dose range would be 1–4 mg/day given in divided doses. When alprazolam is used as an antipanic medication, is often necessary to use a significantly higher dose. In most cases, when these medications are used as antianxiety medications, their use should be restricted to short-term (i.e., 1–2 weeks) for crises or periods of extreme stress. Chronic use has its place, but only rarely and usually only in clients with significant functional disability. Clients should be warned not to drive or use machinery at work until they know how the dose affects them.
2. *As a detoxification agent* in clients addicted to other depressant medications, larger doses of Valium or Librium will be needed; the dosage should then change as the client's clinical condition changes. In alcohol withdrawal, using 50 mg of Librium every two hours is not uncommon. Do not add insult to injury by giving diazepam to someone who is still intoxicated with alcohol or barbiturates. At times, those who are accustomed to a high blood alcohol level can go into withdrawal while still having alcohol in their blood, as long as the blood alcohol level is significantly less than that to which they have become tolerant. In these cases, a benzodiazepine may be indicated to treat the withdrawal.
3. *An acutely out-of-control client* who might be using street

drugs and for whom a good history and diagnosis are not available may have to be sedated when restraints are not enough. In these cases, diazepam 10–20 mg PO may be safer than Thorazine (start low and increase if that is possible). Clients with schizophrenia or mania who are both acutely psychotic and out of control can often be sedated with a combination of an antipsychotic medication and a benzodiazepine. This combination helps reestablish control with a lower dose of antipsychotic medication than would otherwise be necessary, often with fewer side effects.

Diazepam is absorbed faster and more completely by mouth than by intramuscular injection, so it should be given by pill. If a very fast response is required in an emergency situation, lorazepam (Ativan) 2–4 mg can be given by injection. Street drugs are commonly cut with scopolamine or a similar anticholinergic drug that is made worse by Thorazine, and the street drug PCP, or angel dust, can have serious lethal interactions with Thorazine.

Side Effects

1. *All of the benzodiazepines are clearly addictive*, but to put things into perspective, diazepam (Valium) is less addicting and certainly less dangerous than alcohol. The short-acting benzodiazepines, e.g., alprazolam (Xanax), are more addicting than the longer-acting medications in the same class. Medications with a "kick" caused by their rapid onset of action, such as Valium, seem somewhat more subject to abuse than medications with a more gradual onset such as Librium. Anyone who has been taking these medications for more than a few days should have his meds decreased slowly rather than abruptly discontinued. Serious, at times life-threatening, seizures from abrupt withdrawal have been reported with all of the benzodiazepines, but these are more likely with short-acting than long-acting medications. A gradual withdrawal is safer and will also help minimize the inevitable discomfort that accompanies withdrawal.

2. *All of the benzodiazepines may cause drowsiness* (which usually improves after a few days of use). All of these medications also cause a type of intoxication similar to alcohol, with impaired judgment, decreased coordination, light headedness, etc. Clients should be warned about using machinery or driving cars, especially when getting used to these medications. Recent research has suggested that even clients well adjusted to small doses of these medications have a measurable impairment in their driving ability. With short-acting medications, these effects wear off quickly; they remain much longer with the longer-acting medications.
3. *Benzodiazepines can sometimes unleash otherwise inhibited violent behavior.* Again, this "disinhibition" is similar to but much less severe than that with alcohol intoxication.
4. *All of these medications can interfere with memory.* This seems to be a particular problem with triazolam (Halcion) and the other short-acting medications, and with older clients who might already have some memory impairment.

Use during Pregnancy

It has been suggested that these medications might increase birth defects. Although recent reviews have found no evidence of increased birth defect with these medications, as a precaution they should be avoided by pregnant women, especially during the first three months of pregnancy.

Differences among Benzodiazepines

In general, the major differences among benzodiazepines are the speed of onset of action and how long the medication effects last (half-life, or the time it takes for the body to eliminate 50% of the medication). These duration effects vary depending on whether the medication is used occasionally or daily. For the occasional user, Valium's duration is limited by redistribution. Valium rapidly leaves active sites on nerve cells and is absorbed by fat cells. After chronic use, these fat cells become saturated, and duration is limited by the speed with which the medication is broken down by the liver, a much longer process. In the occasional user, Valium is a short-acting medication, but for the chronic user it is a very long-acting medication. Oxazepam (Serax) seems to have a shorter duration of action (half-life) than most of the others. Dalmane has a rapid onset and a long half-life, so, although it is sold as a sleeping pill, it has significant anxiolytic (tranquilizing) action for the next day or two. Both Valium and Librium have moderately long half-lives. The effective half-lives of many medications such as Valium are extended by the presence of active metabolites. That is, the medication is broken down into other chemicals that continue to have sedative and anxiolytic effects.

A benzodiazepine that acts rapidly will be felt by the client as "doing something," while a slower-onset medication is often perceived to be less effective because one does not feel a "kick." On the other hand, rapid-onset sedative hypnotics tend to be more addicting than similar medications with a slower onset of action. When a long-acting medication like Dalmane is given to help with sleep, it can cause a significant hangover the next day, and when given several nights in a row, it can build up in the person and cause tiredness or confusion. A hangover can be avoided by using a very short-acting medication like triazolam. However, when used as a sleeping pill, a short-acting medication can cause the person to wake up partway through the night with rebound insomnia, as the brain reacts to the rapid decrease in medication level.

Alprazolam (Xanax) and clonazepam (Klonopin) are different from the other benzodiazepines in that they appear to have mood-stabilizing properties and are as effective in spontaneous panic attacks as are antidepressants. Clonazepam (Klonopin) is a long-acting, sedating benzodiazepine that is commonly used as an anticonvulsant and may have mood-stabilizing properties as well.

TABLE 11. *Profiles of Common Benzodiazepines*

BENZODIAZEPINES	**Half-life in hours** (including metabolites)	**Daily dosage range (mg)**	**Speed of onset**	**Addiction potential**
alprazolam (Xanax)	9–20	0.5–4	+ +	Higher
chlordiazepoxide (Librium)	28–100	15–100	+ +	Lower
clonazepam (Klonopin)	19–60	1.5–8	+ +	Lower
diazepam (Valium)	30–200	2–40	+ + + +	Higher
flurazepam (Dalmane)	40–250	15–30	+ + +	Moderate
lorazepam (Ativan)	8–24	1–4	+ +	Moderate
oxazepam (Serax)	3–25	30–60	+	Lower
temazepam (Restoril)	3–25	15–30	+ +	Moderate

KEY: + Slow + + Moderate + + + Moderately Fast + + + + Rapid

BUSPIRONE (BUSPAR)

This is a new class of medication that works through an entirely different mechanism of action than either the benzodiazepines or other sedative/hypnotics. It appears to be nonaddictive, not habit-forming, and not subject to abuse (so far). It is the first medication to be anxiolytic (anxiety-reducing) without being sedating. It does not appear to make clients more sensitive to the effects of alcohol or other sedating medications. It is not a muscle relaxant and has no anticonvulsant properties. It is also not useful in helping with alcohol or other drug withdrawal.

Buspirone does appear to have a few idiosyncrasies, which may limit its use in some clients. While Valium and the other benzodiazepines appear to work almost immediately after clients take their first pill, buspirone must be used regularly for up to several weeks before it is fully effective. This means it is best used as a regular medication for someone who can tolerate a delay before it begins working, rather than as a medication with rapid effects that can be taken episodically, as with Valium-type medications.

A second issue has to do with its effectiveness. Double-blind research studies have concluded that BuSpar is as effective as Valium when used by anxious subjects who have never previously used Valium. For some reason, clients who have previously had much experience with Valium or Valium-type medications often feel that BuSpar is less effective. There are at least two possible interpretations to these research findings. One is that the use of Valium-type medications produces long-lasting biological changes in the brain that make BuSpar less effective, and the other is that BuSpar is not really quite as effective as Valium but that it works "well enough" for most people, unless they have already experienced the very powerful and immediate effects of Valium-type medications.

Buspar seems particularly useful for clients who are potential drug abusers and clients who do not like or cannot tolerate the sedative side effects of benzodiazepines.

Sleeping Pills (Hypnotics)

Many clients who complain of insomnia are already sleeping an adequate amount but feel that they "should" be sleeping more or are so bored that they want to sleep more to fill up time. Other clients are concerned that they cannot sleep at night but are taking naps during the day; in these cases the problem is the structure of the sleep cycle rather than a lack of sleep. Other clients are depressed, and the insomnia usually improves when the depression is treated. Some clients with insomnia have a specific sleep disorder, such as sleep apnea. There are specific treatments for some of these disorders, and sleeping pills may actually make things worse.

Sleeping pills are frequently necessary in the hospital because of the noise and strangeness of the hospital and general anxiety of the client. They should never be prescribed automatically, however. They should never be used in a newly admitted client who is still intoxicated (with alcohol or some other depressant) or who still has the obvious after-effects of an overdose. They should be used with caution in older clients who are likely to become confused, disoriented, or (on rare occasions) get a terrifying transient organic psychosis from sleeping pills. Finally, clients with severe respiratory diseases are more apt to develop serious medical complications from the respiratory-depressant side effects of many medications, especially sleeping pills.

When I prescribe sleeping pills for an outpatient, I rarely give more than five pills at a time. It is sometimes nice to have a sleeping pill in the medicine closet for especially bad nights, but it is rarely necessary for anyone to use sleeping pills on a regular basis. Often, the problems caused by sleeping pills are worse than the problems caused by poor sleep.

I do *not* prescribe barbiturates, e.g., secobarbital (Seconal). They are more dangerous and more addicting. Triazolam (Halcion) used to be preferred because of its short half-life and lack of accumulation, especially in the elderly. The concern that triazolam may cause more memory impairment than other medications has led me to avoid it. Tolerance develops to all these medications (with the possible exception of zolpidem). That is, all these medications are less effective for those who take sleeping pills or tranquilizers every day.

The chronic insomnia caused by SSRI antidepressants presents a special problem for some clients. After all of the normal approaches to sleep hygiene have been tried (decrease caffeine, exercise, stop taking naps, do not get up and smoke a cigarette, etc.), using the very sedating antidepressant trazodone is a safe (except for the small risk of priapism) and often effective long-term solution to the problem.

1. *Zolpidem (Ambien)* is a new sleeping pill that seems to have a similar but slightly different mechanism of action than the benzodiazepines. It is reported to be highly effective, non-addicting, and lacking significant side effects. Research suggests that, unlike with the other sleeping pills, tolerance does not develop to zolpidem. This means that zolpidem continues to be effective even when taken nightly for longer periods of time. It is important to remember that the benzodiazepines

were also reported to be non-addicting when they were first introduced, and the particular abuse potential of alprazolam was not initially recognized. At the same time, zolpidem may have some real advantage over other sleeping pills. Ten mg is a typical dose for a healthy adult, and 5 mg is a typical geriatric dose.

2. *Flurazepam (Dalmane)* is very similar to diazepam (Valium) with all of its side effects and advantages. It is rarely lethal in an overdose (unless taken along with alcohol), and it usually provides a comfortable night's sleep with minimum hangover. It is a very long-acting medication, however, with a half-life (including active metabolites) of 40–250 hours. It tends to be longer in older people. This means that half of the medication can remain in the body 4 days after one pill is taken. If a client uses flurazepam every night, the dose from one night is added to the remaining medication from previous nights. This accumulation is a particular problem in elderly clients, who can easily become confused or appear demented as the serum level of flurazepam increases. The usual dose is 15 mg before bedtime.

3. *Temazepam (Restoril)* is a short-acting benzodiazepine that is both safe and effective. The relatively short half-life means that the medication does not accumulate from one night to the next as does flurazepam. The usual dose is 15 mg before bedtime.

4. *Diphenhydramine (Benadryl)* is a sedating antihistamine that can be used as a safe, mild, sleeping medication. The biggest problem with diphenhydramine is its anticholinergic side effects (blocks on the action of acetylcholine). These include dry mouth, constipation, and blurred vision. More importantly, anticholinergic medications like diphenhydramine can also cause confusion, especially in the elderly or in clients who are already taking other anticholinergic medications (including many of the antidepressants or antipsychotic medications). Diphenhydramine has already been mentioned as a treatment

for muscular side effects from antipsychotic medications. The recommended dose is 50–100 mg before bed, with instructions that the client may repeat that dose in one hour. Other sedating antihistamines are also available, including hydroxyzine (Vistaril).

5. *Chloral hydrate* is an old favorite that has long been used because of its relative lack of side effects. It is a more dangerous medication to overdose on than flurazepam. It has a shorter half-life, 7-10 hours, so dose accumulation is less a problem than with flurazepam. Unfortunately, clients become habituated to chloral hydrate fairly rapidly, and after a few days it often becomes less effective. A typical dose is 500 mg before bed for older people and 1,000 mg before bed for young, healthy adults, with an additional 500 mg an hour later if the client still cannot sleep.

6. *Trazodone (Desyrel)* is a sedative antidepressant that can be used as a safe and effective hypnotic, especially for the insomnia caused by SSRI-type antidepressants. A typical dose is 50–400mg before bed. Dry mouth is a common side effect. Priaprism (prolonged, painful erection of the penis) is an uncommon but potentially dangerous side effect in men.

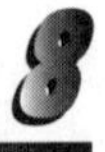

Miscellaneous Medications

Beta-Blockers

Epinephrine and norepinephrine are naturally occurring chemicals within the body that are released by nerve cells and the adrenal gland. They work by stimulating the receptor sites on nerve cells, blood vessels, and other parts of the body. Receptors that are stimulated by epinephrine or norepinephrine are called adrenergic receptors. There are two distinct kinds of receptors called alpha-adrenergic and beta-adrenergic. Beta-blockers, e.g., propranolol (Inderal), simply block these beta receptor sites. These occur throughout the body, which partially explains why these medications are used in conditions that seem unrelated.

Indications for Use

1. *Cardiovascular uses.* Beta-blockers have traditionally been used to help control high blood pressure, treat angina, and control certain kinds of arrhythmias (irregular heartbeats). Beta-blockers are often used to treat migraine headaches, as well as to treat some more unusual conditions associated with an outpouring of epinephrine or norepinephrine.
2. *Tremors.* Benign tremors respond well to these medications. Beta-blockers in low doses are also very effective in treating the tremor that is a common side effect of lithium.
3. *Performance anxiety.* Beta-blockers seem particularly effective in people with performance anxiety. The musician or public

speaker whose anxiety begins to interfere with his or her performance often has a dramatic response to these medications, used in a very low dose. The anticipatory anxiety before the performance is still there, but the specific performance anxiety can be decreased without any sedation or interference with cognitive or motor abilities.

4. *Anxiety with marked somatic (physical) symptoms.* Recently it has been found that beta-blockers block some of the peripheral symptoms of anxiety. The person may still "think" anxious, but these medications can stop the pounding heart, sweaty palms, tremor, etc., that cause the anxiety to feed upon itself and get out of control. These are most useful as antianxiety agents in people who, in fact, have a lot of somatic manifestations of their anxiety.
5. *Akasthisia.* Propranolol is also useful as a treatment for akathisia (the restlessness caused by antipsychotic medications) when the more standard side effect medications are not working.
6. *Violent outbursts.* Some research has suggested that propranolol may be useful in treating certain kinds of violent outbursts, including some of the aggressive behaviors seen in some people with development delay. It also may be useful in treating some schizophrenic clients. The dose range is moderate to high—100–2500 mg/day. Using very high doses may be dangerous, although those dangers are somewhat unclear.

Indications for Use of "Atypical" Beta-Blockers

As was discussed in the beginning of this book, all medications have multiple sites of action. Pindolol (Viskin), an atypical beta-blocker, not only blocks the beta norepinephrine receptor but also blocks serotonin reuptake (and therefore increases serotonin in the synapse). While most beta-blockers can potentiate depressions, pindolol appears to increase the SSRIs' effectiveness in treating depression. It might also accelerate the speed of onset of the antidepressants. A typical dose is 2.5 mg tid. It appears to be less effective with sertraline, probably because of drug-drug interactions.

Side Effects

For the most part, the beta-blockers are very safe medications when used in relatively low doses. They can be extremely dangerous, however, for clients with certain kinds of breathing difficulties. They should never be given to anyone with a history of asthma or chronic, obstructive pulmonary disease. They can also block the clinical recognition of hypoglycemia (low blood sugar). Since people with diabetes may have serious hypoglycemic episodes, the use of beta-blockers for diabetic clients can be dangerous.

The beta-blockers can also cause or potentiate depression, especially in the higher doses used to treat high blood pressure and certain cardiac conditions. They can also cause nightmares and a sense of fatigue.

STIMULANTS

Stimulants, e.g., amphetamine (Dexadrine) and methylphenidate (Ritalin), have had a somewhat checkered career in psychiatry. There are situations where stimulants are clearly useful and safe, but they have been so subject to overuse and abuse that many avoid prescribing them.

Amphetamines

Amphetamines commonly are used with hyperactive children. Stimulants work paradoxically in children (whether hyperactive or not), helping calm them down and increase their attention spans. In normal adults these medications do just the opposite. There is no question that amphetamines are helpful in calming hyperactive children. They help hyperactive children behave more appropriately at home and in school and enable many of these children to stay in normal classes rather than special ed. However, there is ongoing debate about whether hyperactivity is overdiagnosed, and whether many of these children would do better with social/psychological rather than pharmacological intervention.

The use of stimulants in hyperactive adults is receiving increased attention, although the research is still very scanty. Adults who have a clear history of childhood hyperactivity (which is often coupled with some history of learning disability or impulsive behavior) and who continue to have very short attention spans may be helped by stimulants.

Stimulants also have a prominent role in the treatment of resistant depressions. Most depressed clients will respond much better to standard antidepressants, but a small number of depressed clients who have not responded to anything else will respond very well to small amounts of amphetamine. This is indicated only in unusual situations where there is a clear biological component to the depression, when abuse seems unlikely, and when other somatic treatments have been ineffective. The use of stimulants to treat depression in the elderly has recently caught renewed attention. Elderly clients often have major problems with the side effects of typical antidepressants, and stimulants may be a safe and effective alternative for some clients.

Amphetamines are also the medications of choice with narcolepsy.

A typical dose of amphetamine is 5–40 mg/day. Sometimes clients respond well to the drug initially but later develop tolerance, so that the medication loses all effect. Within reason, the dose of the medication can be raised or another stimulant can be tried.

Side Effects. When they are abused, amphetamines cause a "high" or rush that some people find extremely pleasurable. Illicit amphetamines are sold as "speed" and "ice," a new form of crystalline amphetamine that is extremely pure and very potent. When used in high doses, amphetamines can produce a psychosis that resembles paranoid schizophrenia. Even a low dose of amphetamines can cause some individuals to become paranoid. When used in therapeutic doses, amphetamines and other stimulants can cause feelings of anxiety, feeling "wired," and agitated. Amphetamines can also cause problems with sleep, loss of appetite, increased blood pressure, and rapid or irregular pulse. They can cause tics to become worse. There is also concern that the long-term use of stimulants in children may retard normal growth.

Methylphenidate (Ritalin)

Methylphenidate is a stimulant that is less addicting and generally causes fewer side effects than amphetamine. It is most commonly used to treat attention deficit disorder (ADD) in both children and adults. The most common side effects are nervousness and insomnia, although nausea, diarrhea, rashes, increased blood pressure, and increased pulse have been reported. A typical dose of methyphenidate for adults is 20–40 mg a day, but some people require up to 80 mg/day. It is a short-acting medication and typically must be taken two or three times a day.

There is a long-acting form of methylphenidate (Ritalin-SR) that can be given twice a day. The dose of Ritalin-SR is supposed to be the same as regular Ritalin, but anecdotal clinical evidence suggests that a higher dose of the longer-acting preparation may be required to achieve the same effect.

Clonidine (Catapress)

There has been recent interest in using clonidine for posttraumatic stress disorder (PTSD). There is no controlled research, but there have been anecdotal reports and uncontrolled studies suggesting its effectiveness in PTSD commonly seen in refugees of war-torn areas. Clonidine seems to help the hyperarousal and intrusive thoughts common to this disorder. It can be used along with an antidepressant for patients with both PTSD and depression.

Clonidine has also been used to help manage the withdrawal symptoms associated with a number of drugs of abuse, from opiates to cocaine. There is relatively little good data about this use, but clonidine does seem helpful in at least some clients.

Clonidine acts something like norepinephrine in specific nerve cells, and the process decreases the production of real norepinephrine. Clonidine has long been used to lower blood pressure, but recently it has been found to have many other uses. Side effects include dry mouth, tiredness, dizziness, constipation, and skin rashes.

Clonidine is usually started at 0.1 mg once a day, and slowly increased as needed up to a maximum of 0.4–0.6 mg/day in divided doses. It is also available as a patch that lasts for 7 days. It generally takes 2–3 days for someone to get a full serum level after first applying a patch.

Medications Used in the Treatment of Alcohol Dependence

Disulfiram (Antabuse)

Disulfiram can be extremely useful for patients who feel that they cannot control their impulsive use of alcohol. A person will become extremely ill if he consumes alcohol within a few days of taking disulfiram. This means that someone who decides to drink while taking disulfiram must wait up to a week or more before actually taking the first drink. For some people, this period of enforced reflection is extremely useful.

Disulfiram has significant limitations. Many patients refuse to take it or go off it to resume drinking. Some patients can drink even while taking disulfiram, either because they become less ill or because they can get drunk enough to not feel the discomfort caused by the medication. A full disulfiram-alcohol reaction can be dangerous, especially in someone with other serious medical problems, particularly heart disease. Many patients can get a disulfiram-alcohol reaction from cough medicine or even mouthwash containing alcohol. Disulfiram has other significant drug-drug interactions. It can increase the serum level of commonly used medications, such as phenytoin (Dilantin). Disulfiram's side effects include liver disease, rashes, tiredness, headaches, and, at times, psychosis. These side effects are dose-related and are less frequent if the dose is kept at 250 mg/day.

Naltrexone (ReVia)

Naltrexone blocks natural opiate receptors in the brain. It has been used for many years to block the effects of drugs like heroin. For reasons not clearly understood, it also decreases alcohol craving and significantly increases abstinence when it is used as part of a comprehensive alcohol treatment program. Naltrexone is limited to short-term use—generally 3–6 months. There is little apparent benefit from continued use, and there is concern about increasing risk of liver damage with long-term use.

Naltrexone will precipitate sudden, very uncomfortable withdrawal in anyone who has recently used any opiate such as heroin or morphine. Before starting the medication, patients should be asked about opiate use and the risk of withdrawal should be explained. There is also some risk of liver damage, especially at larger doses and perhaps when used over a longer period of time. Naltrexone is usually well tolerated, but it can cause insomnia, anxiety, abdominal pain, nausea, and decreased energy in some patients. A typical dose is 50 mg/day.

Bibliography

Given the rate of change, a newer reference will be more up to date and therefore better than one published a few years ago. I would not buy a general psychopharmacology reference more than two or three years old. I have included some references that are now somewhat out of date but may become available in new editions.

General References for Nonphysicians

Gitlin, M. J. (1996). *The psychotherapist's guide to psychopharmacology* (2nd ed.). New York: Free Press.

This book is designed for the non-physician and is very readable. It includes a lot of clinical wisdom and technical information about medication. It provides a good overview of biological psychiatry, theory, and pharmacology. It is somewhat less useful as a rapid reference book.

Gorman, J. M. (1997). *The essential guide to psychiatric drugs* (3rd ed.). New York: St. Martin's Press.

Available from NAMI, 2101 Wilson Boulevard, Suite 302, Arlington, Virginia 22201. This is an excellent book written for clients, families, and nonmedical professionals. It is very readable and very well organized. It can serve as a detailed reference as questions arise. It contains much more information on more medications than other client-oriented psychopharmacology books.

Yudofsky, S., Hales, R. E., & Ferguson, T. (1991). *What you need to know about psychiatric drugs.* Washington, DC: American Psychiatric Press, Inc.

An excellent general reference book for clients and nonmedical staff, but given the rate of change this is now out of date.

General Psychopharmacology Texts

Gelenberg, A. J., & Bassuk, E. L. (1997). *The practitioner's guide to psychoactive drugs* (4th ed.). New York: Plenum.

An excellent general handbook. This is a brand-new edition and comes highly recommended.

Maxmen, J., & Ward, N. (1996). *Psychotropic drugs: Fast facts* (2nd ed.). New York: Norton.

Schatzberg, A. F., Cole, J. O., & DeBattista, C. (1997). *Manual of clinical psychopharmacology* (3rd ed.). Washington, DC: American Psychiatric Press, Inc.

A very good handbook, very recently updated, and highly recommended.

Werry, J. S., & Aman, M. G. (1993). *Practitioner's guide to psychoactive drugs for children and adolescents.* New York: Plenum.

Medication and Illnesses References for Clients

Greist, J., Jefferson, J., & Marks, I. (1986). *Anxiety and its treatment.* Washington, DC: American Psychiatric Press.

Jefferson, J., & Bohn, M. (1990). *Lithium and manic depression: A guide.* Available from the Lithium Information Center, University of Wisconsin, Department of Psychiatry.

Jefferson, J., & Greist, J. (1990). *Valproate and manic depression: A guide.* Available from the Lithium Information Center, University of Wisconsin, Department of Psychiatry.

Johnston, H. (1990). *Stimulants and hyperactive children: A guide.* Available from the Lithium Information Center, University of Wisconsin, Department of Psychiatry.

Medenwald, J. (1990). *Carbamazepine and manic-depression: A guide.* Available from the Lithium Information Center, University of Wisconsin, Department of Psychiatry.

Weiden, P. J., Scheifler, P. L., Diamond, R. J., Ross, R. (in press). *Switching antipsychotic medications: A guide for consumers and families.* Arlington, Virginia: National Alliance for the Mentally Ill.

This guide provides up-to-date information on the new atypical antipsychotic medications, with an emphasis on how to start one of the new medications and how to switch from a traditional antipsychotic to one of the new medications.

More Specialized Psychopharmacology Texts

Bernstein, J. G. (1995). *Drug therapy in psychiatry* (3rd ed.). St. Louis: Mosby.

This is a good, standard psychopharmacology textbook, well written, well referenced.

Bezchlibnyk-Butler, K. Z., & Jeffries, J. J. (1997). *Clinical handbook of psychotropic drugs* (7th ed.). Kirkland, WA: Hogrefe & Huber.

This manual is a set of charts, tables, and a detailed outline of psychopharmacology. It is excellent for tips and to help organize teaching about psychopharmacology but is less useful as a general text.

Drug facts and comparisons (1997). Published by Facts and Comparisons, 111 West Port Plaza, Suite 300, St. Louis, Missouri, ph: 1-800-223-0554.

This is a compendium of all prescribed medications with indications and side effects, including very useful summary tables. It covers the same material as the *PDR*, but is much more readable. Unfortunately, it is also much more expensive than the *PDR*.

Janicak, P. G., Davis, J. M., Preskorn, S. H., & Ayd, F. J. (1997). *Principles and practice of psychopharmacotherapy* (2nd ed.). Baltimore: Williams & Wilkins.

This is an excellent, very current, highly technical psychopharmacology text. It is very well referenced and includes research support for findings.

Physicians' desk reference (PDR) (50th ed.). (1997).

This book lists every prescription medication marketed in the United States, along with indications, approved dose ranges, and side effects. It has indexes for medications by trade name, by generic name, and by drug category. Unfortunately, it is difficult to interpret information in this book. For example, it lists every reported side effect without giving information about which side effects are common and which have only been reported once, which are serious and which are trivial. *Drug Facts and Comparisons* covers similar information in a more user-friendly format (see above), but the *PDR* is more readily available. The *PDR* is available from Medical Economics, Physicians' Desk Reference, P.O. Box 10689. Des Moines, Iowa 50336.

Schatzberg, A. F., & Nemeroff, C. B. (1995). *Textbook of psychopharmacology*. Washington, DC: American Psychiatric Press, Inc.

This is the current definitive textbook on psychopharmacology.

It is large, detailed, very well referenced, and is very readable. It is also very expensive.

Stahl, S. M. (1996). *Essential psychopharmacology.* New York: Cambridge University Press.

This is an excellent, very readable book on neurotransmitters, receptors, and the basic science of how medications work. It does not discuss specific medications and it is not useful as a clinical guide, but would be highly recommended for someone who wants a more theoretical understanding of psychopharmacology.

Quick and Very Practical Guides

Hyman, S. E., & Tesar, G. E. (Eds.). (1994). *Manual of psychiatric emergencies* (3rd ed.). Boston: Little, Brown.

This is a guide for emergency psychiatry, but it is still very useful and has a lot of practical information about medications. **I highly recommend this book for crisis intervention and emergency psychiatry.**

References on Specific Medications

General Review

Ereshefsky, L., Overman, G. P., & Karp, J. K. (1995, May). Current psychotropic dosing and monitoring guidelines. *Primary Psychiatry,* pp. 42–53.

Antipsychotics

Kane, J. M., Honigfeld, G., Singer, J., Meltzer, H. R., & the Clozaril Collaborative Study Group (1988, Sept.). Clozapine for the treatment-resistant schizophrenic. *Archives of General Psychiatry, 45,* 789–796.

Lieberman, J. A., Kane, J. M., & Johns, C. (1989, Sept.). Clozapine: Guideline for clinical management. *Journal Clinical Psychiatry, 50,* 329–328.

Munetz, M. R., & Benjamin, S. (1988, Nov.). How to examine patients using the abnormal involuntary movement scale. *Journal of Hospital and Community Psychiatry, 39*(11), 1172–1177.

Sullivan, G., & Lukoff, D. (1990, Nov.). Sexual side effects of antipsychotic medication: Evaluation and interventions. *Hospital and Community Psychiatry, 41*(11), 1238–1241.

Antidepressants

Anonymous (1992). Fluoxetine in the treatment of bulimia nervosa: A multicenter, placebo-controlled double-blind trial. Fluoxetine Bulimia Nervousa Collaborative Study Group. *Archives of General Psychiatry, 49*(2), 139–147.

Balon, R. (1995). Effects of antidepressants on human sexuality: Diagnosis and management. *Primary Psychiatry* 2(8).

Gelenberg, A. (1990, March). Update: The MAOI diet. *Biological Therapies in Psychiatry Newsletter, 15*(3).

Gelenberg, P. (1995, Aug.). The P450 family. *Biological Therapies in Psychiatry Newsletter, 18*(8).

Markovitz, P. J., Calabrese, J. R., Schulz, S.C., & Meltzer, H. Y. (1991). Fluoxetine in the treatment of borderline and schizotypal personality disorders. *American Journal of Psychiatry, 148,* 1064–1067.

Shulman, K. I., Walker, J. E., MacKenzie, S., & Knowles, S. (1989, Dec.). Dietary restriction, tyramine, and the use of monoamine oxidase inhibitors. *Journal of Clinical Psychopharmacology, 9*(6), 397–402.

Lithium

Gitlin, M. J. (1993). Lithium-induced renal insufficiency. *Journal of Psychopharmacology, 13*(4).

Anxiolytics

Griffiths, R. R., & Wolf, W. (1990, Aug.). Relative abuse liability of different benzodiazepines in drug abusers. *Journal of Clinical Psychopharmacology, 10*(4), 237–243.

Miscellaneous

Kinzie, J. D., & Leung, P. (1989). Clonidine in Cambodian patients with posttraumatic stress disorder. *Journal of Nervous and Mental Disease, 177*(9).

Newsletters

Gelenberg, A. (Ed.). *Biological therapies in psychiatry newsletter.* St. Louis: Mosby Year Book.

Primary psychiatry: MBL Communications.
This is a journal oriented toward family practice and other pri-

mary care physicians. It has excellent reviews of basic psychopharmacology, with extremely useful charts and very good summaries of current medications. It is practical, and despite its focus on physicians is very readable. It is available free of charge for primary care physicians. Psychiatrists can also request a subscription.

Roche, J. (Ed.). *Psychiatry drug alerts.* MJ Powers.

Computer-Based Drug Interaction Program

A good, inexpensive, computer-based program for drug-drug interactions is published by the Medical Letter. It is available for approximately $100 for initial program and 4 updates.

Web Sites

http://uhs.bsd.uchicago.edu/dr-bob/tips/tips.html

My favorite psychopharmacology web site is the Psychopharmacology Tips page, which is an indexed archive of the psychopharmacology discussion group. It provides information about current innovative uses of medications, recognition and treatment of side effects, and is a repository of cutting edge information. It is based on the contributors' clinical experience, not on research, and it must be used with this in mind.

http://www.mentalhealth.com/p.30.html

A web page of pharmacology references that provides basic information about prescribed medication.

http://uhs.bsd.uchicago.edu/scrs/uspdi.html

Drug information leaflets for patients, prepared by the US Pharmacopia. You can search for and get very basic information about any prescription medication. The psychotropic medications are listed by type to make them very easy to find.

http://www.nami.org/

Web page for the National Alliance for the Mentally Ill.

http://freenet.msp.mn.us/ip/stockley/mental_health.html

A good general starting place for finding mental health resources on the Internet.

http://www.samhsa.gov/

Substance Abuse and Mental Health Association (SAMHSA)

Drug Indentification by Brand Name

Brand Name	Generic Name	Chief Action
Akineton	biperiden	Antiparkinsonian, anticholinergic
Ambiem	zolpidem	Sleeping pill
Amytal	amobarbital	Sleeping pill, barbiturate
Anafranil	clomipramine	Tricyclic antidepressant—used with OCD
Antabuse	disulfiram	Anti-alcohol
Artane	trihexyphenidyl	Antiparkinsonian, anticholinergic
Asendin	amoxapine	Tricyclic antidepressant
Atarax	hydroxyzine	Sedating antihistamine
Ativan	lorazepam	Antianxiety, benzodiazepine
Atropine Sulfate	atropine	Anticholinergic
Benadryl	diphenhydramine	Sedating antihistamine
BuSpar	buspirone	Antianxiety
Butisol	butabarbital	Antianxiety, barbiturate
Catapres	clonidine	Alpha adrenergic agonist
Clozaril	clozapine	Atypical antipsychotic
Cogentin	benztropine	Antiparkinsonian, anticholinergic
Cylert	pemoline	Stimulant
Dalmane	flurazepam	Sleeping pill, benzodiazepine
Depakene	valproic acid	Anticonvulsant, mood stabilizer
Depakote	divalproex	Anticonvulsant, mood stabilizer
Desyrel	trazodone	Sedating antidepressant
Dexedrine	dextroamphetamine	Stimulant
Doral	quazepam	Sleeping pill
Doriden	glutethimide	Sleeping pill (no longer used)
Effexor	venlafaxine	New generation antidepressant
Elavil	amitriptyline	Tricyclic antidepressant
Eldepryl	selegiline	MAOI used for Parkinson's disease
Equanil	meprobamate	Antianxiety (older medication)
Eskalith	lithium	Mood stabilizer
Fastin	phentermine	Appetite suppressant
Halcion	triazolam	Sleeping pill, benzodiazepine
Haldol	haloperidol	Antipsychotic
Inapsine	droperidol	Antipsychotic (used in anesthesia)

Brand Name	Generic Name	Chief Action
Inderal	propranolol	Beta blocker
Janimine	imipramine	Tricyclic antidepressant
Kemadrin	procyclidine	Antiparkinson, anticholinergic
Klonopin	clonazepam	Antianxiety, benzodiazepine
Lamactil	lamotrigine	Anticonvulsant, mood stabilizer
Larodopa	levodopa	Dopamine booster used for Parkinson's disease
Librium	chlordiazepoxide	Antianxiety, benzodiazepine
Lithane	lithium	Mood stabilizer
Lithobid	lithium	Mood stabilizer
Loxitane	loxapine	Antipsychotic
Ludiomil	maprotiline	Antidepressant
Luvox	fluvoxamine	SSRI antidepressant
Marplan	isocarboxazid	MAOI antidepressant (no longer marketed)
Mellaril	thioridazine	Antipsychotic
Miltown	meprobamate	Antianxiety (older medication)
Moban	molindone	Antipsychotic
Narcan	naloxone	Narcotic antagonist
Nardil	phenelzine	MAOI antidepressant
Navane	thiothixene	Antipsychotic
Neurotin	gabapentin	Anticonvulsant, mood stabilizer
Noctec	chloral hydrate	Sleeping pill
Norpramin	desipramine	Tricyclic antidepressant
Orap	pimozide	Antipsychotic
Pamelor	nortriptyline	Tricyclic antidepressant
Paral	paraldehyde	Sleeping pill
Parlodel	bromocriptine	Dopamine agonist used for side effects
Parnate	tranylcypromine	MAOI antidepressant
Paxil	paroxetine	SSRI antidepressant
Placidyl	ethchlorvynol	Sleeping pill
Pondimin	fenfluramine	Appetite supressant
Prolixin	fluphenazine	Antipsychotic
ProSom	estazolam	Sleeping pill
Prozac	fluoxetine	SSRI antidepressant
Remeron	mirtazepine	New generation antidepressant
Restoril	temazepam	Sleeping pill, benzodiazepine
ReVia	naltrexone	Narcotic antagonist
Risperdal	risperidone	Atypical antipsychotic
Ritalin	methylphenidate	Stimulant
Seconal	secobarbital	Sleeping pill, barbiturate (dangerous)
Serax	oxazepam	Antianxiety, benzodiazepine
Serentil	mesoridazine	Antipsychotic
Seroquel	quetiapine	Atypical antipsychotic
Serzone	nefazodone	New generation antidepressant
Sinemet	carbidopa-levodopa	Dopamine booster for Parkinson's disease

Brand Name	Generic Name	Chief Action
Sinequan	doxepine	Tricyclic antidepressant
Stelazine	trifluoperazine	Antipsychotic
Surmontil	trimipramine	Tricyclic antidepressant
Symmetrel	amantadine	Antiparkinson
Tegretol	carbamazepine	Mood stabilizer, anticonvulsant
Thorazine	chlorpromazine	Antipsychotic
Tofranil	imipramine	Tricyclic antidepressant
Tranxene	clorazepate	Antianxiety, benzodiazepine
Trilafon	perphenazine	Antipsychotic
Valium	diazepam	Antianxiety, benzodiazepine
Vistaril	hydroxyzine	Sedating antihistamine
Vivactil	protriptyline	Tricyclic antidepressant
Wellbutrin	buproprion	New generation antidepressant
Xanax	alprazolam	Antianxiety, benzodiazepine
Zeldox	ziprasidone	Atypical antipsychotic
Zyprexa	olanzapine	Atypical antipsychotic

Drug Identification by Generic Name

Generic Name	Brand Name	Chief Action
alprazolam	Xanax	Antianxiety
amantadine	Symmetrel	Antiparkinson
amitriptyline	Elavil	Tricyclic antidepressant
amobarbital	Amytal	Sleeping pill, barbiturate
amoxapine	Asendin	Tricyclic antidepressant
atropine	Atropine Sulfate	Anticholinergic
benztropine	Cogentin	Antiparkinson, anticholinergic
biperiden	Akineton	Antiparkinson, anticholinergic
bromocriptine	Parlodel	Dopamine agonist used for side effects
buproprion	Wellbutrin	New generation antidepressant
buspirone	BuSpar	Antianxiety
butabarbital	Butisol	Antianxiety, barbiturate
carbamazepine	Tegretol	Mood stabilizer, anticonvulsant
carbidopa-levodopa	Sinemet	Dopamine booster used for Parkinson's disease
chloral hydrate	Noctec	Sleeping pill
chlordiazepoxide	Librium	Antianxiety, benzodiazepine
chlorpromazine	Thorazine	Antipsychotic
clomipramine	Anafranil	Tricyclic antidepressant—used with OCD
clonazepam	Klonopin	Antianxiety, benzodiazepine
clonidine	Catapres	Alpha adrenergic agonist
clorazepate	Tranxene	Antianxiety, benzodiazepine
clozapine	Clozaril	Atypical antipsychotic
desipramine	Norpramin	Tricyclic antidepressant
dextroamphetamine	Dexedrine	Stimulant
diazepam	Valium	Antianxiety, benzodiazepine
diphenhydramine	Benadryl	Sedating antihistamine
disulfiram	Antabuse	Anti-alcohol
divalproex	Depakote	Anticonvulsant, mood stabilizer
doxepine	Sinequan	Tricyclic antidepressant
droperidol	Inapsine	Antipsychotic (used in anesthesia)
estazolam	ProSom	Sleeping pill
ethchlorvynol	Placidyl	Sleeping pill

Generic Name	Brand Name	Chief Action
fenfluramine	Pondimin	Appetite supressant
fluoxetine	Prozac	SSRI antidepressant
fluphenazine	Prolixin	Antipsychotic
flurazepam	Dalmane	Sleeping pill, benzodiazepine
fluvoxamine	Luvox	SSRI antidepressant
gabapentin	Neurotin	Anticonvulsant, mood stabilizer
glutethimide	Doriden	Sleeping pill (no longer used)
haloperidol	Haldol	Antipsychotic
hydroxyzine	Atarax, Vistaril	Sedating antihistamine
imipramine	Tofranil, Janimine	Tricyclic antidepressant
isocarboxazid	Marplan	MAOI antidepressant (no longer marketed)
lamotrigine	Lamactil	Anticonvulsant, mood stabilizer
levodopa	Larodopa	Dopamine booster used for Parkinson's disease
lithium	Eskalith, Lithane, Lithobid	Mood stabilizer
lorazepam	Ativan	Antianxiety, benzodiazepine
loxapine	Loxitane	Antipsychotic
maprotiline	Ludiomil	Antidepressant
meprobamate	Miltown, Equanil	Antianxiety (older medication)
mesoridazine	Serentil	Antipsychotic
methylphenidate	Ritalin	Stimulant
mirtazepine	Remeron	New generation antidepressant
molindone	Moban	Antipsychotic
naloxone	Narcan	Narcotic antagonist
naltrexone	ReVia	Narcotic antagonist
nefazodone	Serzone	New generation antidepressant
nortriptyline	Pamelor	Tricyclic antidepressant
olanzapine	Zyprexa	Atypical antipsychotic
oxazepam	Serax	Antianxiety, benzodiazepine
paraldehyde	Paral	Sleeping pill
paroxetine	Paxil	SSRI antidepressant
pemoline	Cylert	Stimulant
perphenazine	Trilafon	Antipsychotic
phenelzine	Nardil	MAOI antidepressant
phentermine	Fastin	Appetite suppressant
pimozide	Orap	Antipsychotic
procyclidine	Kemadrin	Antiparkinson, anticholinergic
propranolol	Inderal	Beta blocker
protriptyline	Vivactil	Tricyclic antidepressant
quazepam	Doral	Sleeping pill
quetiapine	Seroquel	Atypical antipsychotic
risperidone	Risperdal	Atypical antipsychotic
secobarbital	Seconal	Sleeping pill, barbiturate (dangerous)
selegiline	Eldepryl	MAOI used for Parkinson's disease
temazepam	Restoril	Sleeping pill, benzodiazepine

Generic Name	Brand Name	Chief Action
thioridazine	Mellaril	Antipsychotic
thiothixene	Navane	Antipsychotic
tranylcypromine	Parnate	MAOI antidepressant
trazodone	Desyrel	Sedating antidepressant
triazolam	Halcion	Sleeping pill, benzodiazepine
trifluoperazine	Stelazine	Antipsychotic
trihexyphenidyl	Artane	Antiparkinson, anticholinergic
trimipramine	Surmontil	Tricyclic antidepressant
valproic acid	Depakene	Anticonvulsant, mood stabilizer
venlafaxine	Effexor	New generation antidepressant
ziprasidone	Zeldox	Atypical antipsychotic
zolpidem	Ambiem	Sleeping pill

Index